OXFORD MEDICAL PUBLICATIONS

Ethics and the Law in Intensive Care

Ethics and the Law in Intensive Care

Edited by

N. PACE

Consultant Anaesthetist, Western Infirmary, Glasgow

and

SHEILA A. M. McLEAN

International Bar Association Professor of Law and Ethics in Medicine, and Director of the Institute of Law and Ethics in Medicine, University of Glasgow

OXFORD   NEW YORK   MELBOURNE   TORONTO
OXFORD UNIVERSITY PRESS
1996

Oxford University Press, Walton Street, Oxford OX2 6DP

Oxford   New York
Athens   Auckland   Bangkok   Bombay
Calcutta   Cape Town   Dar es Salaam   Delhi
Florence   Hong Kong   Istanbul   Karachi
Kuala Lumpur   Madras   Madrid   Melbourne
Mexico City   Nairobi   Paris   Singapore
Taipei   Tokyo   Toronto

and associated companies in
Berlin   Ibadan

Oxford is a trade mark of Oxford University Press

Published in the United States
by Oxford University Press Inc., New York

A catalogue record for this book is available from the British Library

Library of Congress Cataloging in Publication Data

Ethics and the law in intensive care / edited by N. Pace and
Sheila A.M. McLean.
p. cm.—(Oxford medical publications)
Includes index.
ISBN 0 19 262520 9
1. Critical care medicine—Moral and ethical aspects. 2. Critical
care medicine—Law and legislation. I. Pace, N. (Nicholas A.)
II. McLean, Sheila. III. Series
[DNLM: 1. Ethics, Medical. 2. Intensive Care. W 50 E8412 1996]
RC86.95.E845   1996
174'.2—dc20
DNLM/DLC
for Library of Congress   95–33647
                                                                  CIP

Typeset by Palimpsest Book Production Limited,
Polmont, Stirlingshire
Printed in Great Britain by Bookcraft Ltd,
Midsomer Norton, Bath, Avon

Preface

The aim of this book is to provide readers with an insight into the many complex ethical and legal dilemmas health care staff regularly encounter when working in an intensive care unit. The intensive care unit is different in many respects from the normal general medical ward. Patients are more ill, usually unconscious, and their lives are maintained by means of the most complex technology. Furthermore, the rapid advances made in this medical technology have meant that doctors today are frequently capable of keeping most patients alive, sometimes for very long periods of time. However, the greater availability and use of technology has created ethical, legal, and economic dilemmas that were unthinkable only a few years ago. Today the question is frequently not whether such a patient *can* be treated but whether treatment *should* be started or continued. Unfortunately, in many cases, the ITU staff concerned may be uncertain about the ethical issues raised and very frequently have no idea of the current attitude of the law. This is clearly exemplified by their approach to obtaining consent when an unconscious, and hence legally incompetent, patient requires medical intervention. The current practice of obtaining consent from relatives has no foundation in law, except in very limited situations, such as when the patient is a minor. It should further be pointed out that in many areas of medicine the law is non existent and hence may need to be deduced from various legal principles. Because much of the law is undeveloped in the UK, frequent reference will be made to cases in other jurisdictions.

There are a great number of health care staff who are regularly involved in the management of patients in an intensive care unit. In view of the fact that medical practice is becoming much more of a team matter, all members of this team, such as medical staff, nursing staff, physiotherapists, etc. need an understanding of the various issues raised as they are directly involved in decision making. This book is aimed primarily at them, although it has been written in such a way that any non-medically trained person will gain an understanding of the many dilemmas raised. Although the occasional anecdotal reference may be made, the book is not a collection of case histories. Rather, the aim of the book is to provoke discussion based upon analysis of certain principles. Indeed, since it is anticipated that in many cases the reader will have no prior knowledge of ethics or law, the authors have been requested to explain fully ethical or legal principles where necessary. Readers will, therefore, be allowed to make up their own minds about what is ethically correct in the various situations, such as withdrawing treatment from patients in a persistent vegetative state or electively ventilating patients solely for later use of their organs. It is indeed unfortunate that very little time is spent during training discussing the various issues that regularly crop up during every day's working practice in the ITU. Staff are left to muddle through, coming to a conclusion that is not based on any sound ethical or legal principle. Frequently, decisions are reached by consensus. The dissenter in fact is usually viewed as a trouble maker.

This book should provide the reader with a sound basis for the conceptual analysis of some of modern medicines most complex and difficult decisions.

Glasgow   N. P.
November 1995   S. McL.

Contents

Contributors

Malcolm G. Booth
Consultant Anaesthetist, Royal Infirmary, Glasgow G4 0SF.

R.S. Downie
Professor of Moral Philosophy, University of Glasgow, Glasgow G12 8QQ.

G.R. Dunstan
Professor Emeritus of Moral and Social Theology, University of London, 9 Maryfield Avenue, Pennsylvania, Exeter EX4 6JN.

Roger Dyson
Honorary Professor and Director, Clinical Management Unit, Centre for Health Planning and Management, Darwin Building, Keele University, Staffordshire ST5 5SR.

Michael Heap
Registrar, Department of Anaesthetics, Norfolk and Norwich Hospital, Brunswick Road, Norwich NR1 3SR, UK.

Sydney Jacobs
Department of Anaesthesia, Riyadh al Kharj Hospital, PO Box 7897, Riyadh 11159, Kingdom of Saudi Arabia.

Bryan Jennett
Professor Emeritus of Neurosurgery, Department of Neurosurgery, Southern General Hospital, Glasgow G51 4TF.

J.K. Mason
Regius Professor (Emeritus) of Forensic Medicine, and Honorary Fellow, Faculty of Law, University of Edinburgh, Edinburgh EH8 9YL.

Lesley McTurk
Chief Executive Officer, Mercy Hospital and Health Services, 98 Mountain Road, Epsom, Auckland, New Zealand.

Kath M. Melia
Senior Lecturer and Head of Department of Nursing Studies, Adam Ferguson Building, 40 George Square, University of Edinburgh, Edinburgh EH8 9LL.

N.S. Morton
Consultant in Paediatric Anaesthesia and Intensive Care, Royal Hospital for Sick Children, and Honorary Clinical Senior Lecturer, University of Glasgow, Glasgow G3 8SJ.

Saxon A. Ridley
Consultant in Anaesthesia and Intensive Care, Consultant in Charge of Intensive Care Unit, Norfolk and Norwich Hospital, Brunswick Road, Norwich NR1 3SR.

Peter G.M. Wallace
Director, Anaesthesia and Intensive Care, Western Infirmary, Glasgow G11 6NT.

Introduction to Medical Ethics

R.S. Downie

1. Introduction

In recent years health care professionals, and the public they serve, have become more conscious of the complexity of the moral problems that can be created by caring for other people. There is now growing awareness of the need to identify clearly what these moral problems are, and to arrive at possible solutions for the patients and for the nurses, doctors, or other professionals concerned, while taking into account wider social issues.

An initial complication is that problems in health care have traditionally been identified as 'ethical' rather than 'moral' and there has developed the mistaken idea that there are special kinds of expertise called 'medical ethics' and 'nursing ethics', and correspondingly, that those who care for others have special claims to knowing or deciding what is right and wrong in health and illness. Moreover, by being members of a profession concerned with people's well-being, doctors in particular, but also nurses and other health care workers, have allowed themselves to be seen as arbiters in public and private moral dilemmas for which they may have no more expertise than any other thoughtful and considerate person. On the other hand, those who care for others do have special kinds of non-moral knowledge and they also have the experience of dealing with those who are seriously ill. That knowledge and experience gives them some claim to be listened to, and it will certainly affect their moral or ethical decisions. What would be helpful is that those who care for us when we are ill should have some familiarity with the arguments and concepts which are employed in ethical discussion.

There is a second source of confusion which must be removed at the start—the term 'ethics' is ambiguous. First, 'ethics' can refer to that branch of philosophy also called 'moral philosophy'. Ethics in this sense is a theoretical study of practical morality and its aim is to discover, analyse, and relate to each other the fundamental concepts and principles of ordinary practical morality.

The second main sense of 'ethics' is ordinary morality or value judgements as they are found in a professional context. This usage brings out the *continuity* between the moral problems of everyday life and those encountered in hospitals or other spheres of professional practice. Morality or ethics must be seen broadly as including the whole area of value judgements about good and harm.

The third sense of 'ethics' refers to codes of procedure, or ethics narrowly conceived. These are important for they provide some of the principles that underlie professional activity and they apply across cultural and national boundaries.

It is worthwhile stressing the difference between the second broad sense of ethics as value judgements and the narrow sense, which refers simply to the items on a traditional list. For example, in the broad sense it is a moral or value judgement that a given patient, all factors considered, ought to be allowed home despite the risk of a recurrence of his or her problem. However, clearly this decision does not raise a question of morality or ethics narrowly conceived. It is because many health care professions take ethics or morality in the narrow sense that they are unaware of the extent to which they are continually making moral or value judgements in the broad sense. There are certainly technical—scientific and social—factors involved in deciding whether or not a given patient ought to be allowed home. But the decision about what in the end ought to be done goes beyond the technical and encompasses the professional's overall judgement as to what is for the total good of the patient. This overall judgement, all things considered, of the patient's good is what I mean by a moral or value judgement. One of the central aims of teaching ethics is to make the professional aware of the all-pervasive nature of such value judgements and the extent to which the professional's own values affect decisions.

2. Doctors' duties

From the time of Hippocrates until the 1960s medical ethics was seen in terms of doctors' duties to patients. These duties have traditionally been thought of as those of not harming the patient (non-maleficence) and of helping the patient (beneficence). Underlying these two apparently simple types of duty there are, however, complexities. Medical understanding of these duties has been affected by three different currents of thinking. Let us examine these currents, which are also discussed by Jonsen.[1]

The first current is the one flowing from the origins of modern medicine in the Ancient Greek world. When the Hippocratic Oath requires the physician not to harm but to help, it is against a background of Greek craftsmanship. The art or craft (*techne*) of the carpenter is to work on wood according to the nature of wood. There are bounds or limits concerning what is appropriate for each craft, and to go beyond these bounds is to be guilty of *hubris* or pride. Hence, when the Greek doctor promises not to harm and to do good to the patient, what is intended is much the same requirement as that laid on the carpenter when, as a good craftsman, he tries not to damage his material, wood, but rather to bring out its nature as wood. We might term the Hippocratic ethic that of the competent craftsman. The relevant portion of the Hippocratic Oath really indicates that there are constraints on the skill or art of medicine; it does not truly involve beneficence in our modern sense. However, beneficence in our modern sense enters the scene via the Samaritan tradition in medicine. It is known that St. Luke was a physician and there is some evidence that the Good Samaritan was meant to be a physician—certainly he treated the man fallen by the wayside with an infundation of oil and wine, which was a remedy for wounds in Greek medicine. However that may be, the ideal of the Good Samaritan, as one who ministers to the sick despite inconvenience and danger to himself, was one which enormously affected the tradition of medicine, and it gave us the ideal of beneficence in something like its modern form. Even so, not completely like its form in modern medicine, because another current also affected medical beneficence. Historians of medicine have debated the origins of this tradition, and it may have been in the religious orders that were founded to care for the sick and wounded during the Crusades. For example, the Order of Knights Hospitallers was founded in the eleventh century to provide hostels for pilgrims to the Holy Land and to care for the sick, and later for those wounded in the Crusades. The members of this Order came mainly from noble families and were dedicated to serve 'our lords, the sick' (a favourite phrase). This tradition continued in the religious orders, and it emerged in a different form in the eighteenth century when the status and education of doctors began once again to improve, and the image of the gentleman-physician began to reappear. The opening words of the influential book on medical ethics, written by the British physician Thomas Percival (1803),[2] bear witness in elegant language to the ethic of *noblesse oblige*:

Physicians and surgeons should minister to the sick, reflecting that the ease, health and lives of those committed to their charge depend on their skills, attention and fidelity. They should study, in their deportment, so to unite tenderness with steadiness, and condescension with authority, as to inspire the minds of their patients with gratitude, respect and confidence.

These words echo the sentiments of the Knights Hospitallers of the Crusades, and they were incorporated into the Code of Ethics of the American Medical Association and stood unchanged from 1847 to 1912; as Jonsen says (p. 66), their spirit lived long after that.

To conclude, we can say that all doctors would nowadays subscribe to the ethical idea that they have duties not to harm and to do good to their patients, but they may be unaware of the fact that the medical interpretation of these duties has been coloured by (at least) three traditions: the Hippocratic tradition of competent craftsmanship, the Good Samaritan tradition of helping one's neighbour in all circumstances, and the Knights' Hospitaller tradition of noble service.

This rich medical ethos, which I shall call the 'main tradition', remained largely undisturbed from the Greek world to the end of the 1950s. Since then, however, there have been at least three attacks on it, deriving from three different sets of ideas: the emergence of nursing as an independent profession and along with that the development of a team approach to health care; the rise of patients' rights movements; and the need for rationing, following the growth of demand on medical services. These movements overlap in various ways, and all are particular manifestations of broader social changes.

3. Teams and the nursing profession

The demand for a team approach to health care has been greatly influenced by the rise of nursing to full professional status. Nurses are nowadays very intolerant of the traditional references of doctors to 'my' patients. They are increasingly demanding consultation before important decisions affecting patient care are taken. Hence, we have one partial explanation of the increasing use of teams making joint decisions. Other parts of the explanation—such as the increasingly technical complexity of the decisions that require a range of specialist opinions—do not concern us here. But granted that nursing opinion is increasingly important in decisions we find the beginnings of a new approach to health care that involves more group decisions. The emergence of group decision-making (and the extent of it varies a great deal) is therefore a challenge to the older ideas of the doctors' duties. Let us hope that if there can be broad discussions involving not only different specialists but also different gender perspectives, more balanced decisions may result.

Before leaving this topic, however, we should note that group decision-making involves group responsibility. If the nursing profession wants an equal claim to be heard, then nurses must be willing to be held responsible for their decisions.

Although the rise of other professional groups, and the consequent challenge to male medical supremacy in decision-making, has perhaps been psychologically disturbing to the medical profession, there is no reason why it cannot be assimilated into the traditional approach to patient care. Instead of thinking of the supremacy of medical duties to patients we can think of team-based duties and hope that the decisions of a broadly based team are more balanced and less 'gung-ho' then they otherwise might have been. This is a development and humanizing of the 'main tradition' rather than an abandonment of it.

4. Patients' rights and autonomy

A more radical challenge to the tradition arises from from the appearance of the patients' rights movement. This movement is not unconnected with the rise of nursing as a profession because many nurses see themselves as being 'the patient's advocate', and support their patients' rights. However, this movement is also influenced by many other considerations. One broad influence has been the general democratization of society in the post-war period. In general terms, the public require involvement in decisions that are going to affect them. This move to more openness and consultation has affected medicine as much as any other branch of society. More specifically, within medicine, the rise of patients' rights movements was influenced by the exposure of abuses in medical research, when it emerged in the 1960s that, in some cases, informed consent was not being obtained for dangerous research. The result was that, first in the US and then in the UK, research ethics committees were established and this in turn influenced the medical approach to the doctor–patient relationship.

The concept that has been adopted to encapsulate the idea of the rights of patients is 'autonomy'. Codes of medical ethics and philosophical discussion from the 1970s onwards increasingly added 'respect for the patient's autonomous decisions' to the duties of non-maleficence and beneficence. At about the same time the concept of 'justice' was brought into play. For example, treating individual patients justly, by observing their rights, and entitlement of *all* patients to equal shares in the distribution of health care. For almost two decades, discussions of medical ethics have been conducted in the US and the UK very largely in terms of the four principles of non-maleficence, beneficence, respect for autonomy, and justice; and many influential textbooks have been written, and indeed are still being written, using them as the essential principles of humane discussion in medical ethics.

Before going on to examine the principle of respect for autonomy in more detail we should perhaps elaborate the philosophical position. The four principles can be seen, and were seen by the majority of writers, as first-order moral principles, to be used in reaching medical decisions when ethical questions were raised. It is a separate matter, and one for the moral philosopher, how these principles can be justified. Are they each an expression of a single underlying principle or are they each independently valid, and if so what happens if they clash? These and many related matters are the concern of moral philosophy proper, and I do not intend to pursue them in this short introduction to medical ethics. However, it is worth noting because the terms are often used in ethical debate, and those who think that there is a single underlying principle often identify that principle as the principle of utility—that actions are right if they maximize individual preferences, or, in older terminology, if they bring about the greatest happiness of the greatest number. As opposed to the utilitarians, those who hold that the principles can each independently be seen to be valid have been called deontologists. However, I shall not pursue the interesting debates which have clustered round these theories.

Returning to the principle of respect for the patient's autonomy we shall find that once we look beyond this maxim it is not clear what is meant by 'autonomy'. There are, in fact, at least two ways of interpreting it. One interpretation is compatible with the 'main tradition' of medical ethics and is an enrichment of it ('preference autonomy'), but the second ('consumer autonomy') is not compatible, and indeed it implies a radical change in the doctor–patient relationship.

The idea of 'autonomy', of persons as self-determining, self-governing beings, is first discussed with a proper understanding of what it means by Kant. He assumes that people are essentially rational, although our desires may at times blind us. Decisions that are made as a result of dominant or blinding desires he called 'heteronomous'. They are not truly the desires of the self, for they are caused by the non-rational aspects of human nature. The Kantian tradition of moral philosophy as it affected medical ethics was modified by the liberal tradition of John Stuart Mill. Briefly, Mill argues that we have a right to do whatever we want unless it can be shown that we are harming others. The key difference between Kant's approach to autonomy and Mill's lies in the respective emphases given to rationality and preferences. For Kant, a decision is autonomous if it is rational (whether it expresses our preferences or not). For Mill, an autonomous decision does express our preference and it is less important whether the decision is rational. These traditions have merged and what developed is that 'autonomy' is the expression of informed preferences or consent to whatever we do, or is done to us by others.

This fused Kantian–Millean conception of autonomy, as preference or as informed consent, is one that can be absorbed by the 'main tradition'. No doubt the doctor–patient relationship always involved some sort of consultation and discussion, and we can interpret the more recent emphasis on autonomy—on obtaining informed consent for all medical decisions—as an extension of and an insistence on that process of consultation. It can be seen as an antidote to the paternalism which was the pathology of the doctor–patient relationship in the past, and as a way of modernizing the relationship, of modifying it in terms of the modern ethos of openness in human relationships. It is important to note, however, that autonomous choices or informed consent in this sense take place within the context of a professional consultation, with the patient retaining the right of veto to unwanted treatment and the doctor retaining the right of veto to treatment professionally considered useless or harmful. However, let us look at the important difference when 'preference autonomy' becomes 'consumer autonomy'.

To set the scene, consider a genuine situation of consumer autonomy. Suppose that I go into a shoe shop and ask for a pair of strong shoes for walking along country lanes. I try on various pairs which do not appeal to me and then my eye lights on a pair of shiny patent leather shoes and I say I want to buy them. A good salesperson will explain to me that they are not appropriate shoes for my purposes, but if I insist that these are the ones I want the salesperson has no obligation to refuse the sale, having advised against it. I am here exercising consumer autonomy. Can this idea be carried over into the medical context? Many ethicists think that it can, and indeed the British Government is encouraging the idea of consumer autonomy in health care to the extent that patients are being exhorted to see themselves as customers. Let us look at the ethics literature on this.

Take the situation in which a patient, or relatives of the patient, request treatment which the doctor believes is useless or even harmful. In a study surveying the literature on this, Paris *et al.*[3] note that doctors will almost always continue treatment if requested by patients or relatives even if they regard it as futile. They do this because they believe that patient autonomy carries with it the right to whatever treatment the patient requests. Moreover, this view is supported by many US ethicists. For example, Veatch and Spicer (1992) maintain that a physician is obliged to supply requested treatment even if the request 'deviates intolerably' from established standards or is in terms of the doctor's judgement 'grossly inappropriate'.[4]

In discussion of this we should note, first, that Veatch and Spicer, and many other US ethicists who hold this view of patient autonomy, are surely mistaken if they think that it follows from any interpretation of the doctrine of autonomy that people should be given something simply on the grounds that they demand it.

Secondly, we must remember that the principle of respect for autonomy applies not only to the patient but also to the doctor, and if in the doctor's professional opinion the requested treatment is 'grossly inappropriate' then the doctor has no duty to provide it; indeed, he has a duty *not* to provide it. This position has, in fact, been supported by the English Court of Appeal. In a case in which a physician had indicated that he would not concur with a family's request to give a dying patient ventilatory treatment if that became necessary to sustain the patient's life, Lord Justice Donaldson stated that 'courts should not require a medical practitioner . . . to adopt a course of treatment which in the *bona fide* clinical judgement of the practitioner was contraindicated'. Lord Justice Balcome went further and wrote that he 'could conceive of no situation where it would be proper to order a doctor to treat a patient in a manner contrary to his or her clinical judgement'. In other words, the Court of Appeal is here supporting the professional autonomy of the doctor.[5]

Thirdly, let us consider the change in ethos or culture that is leading to the consumer view of autonomy, and the implications of the change for the 'main tradition' of the doctor–patient relationship. It will be remembered that in a true consumer situation the shoe salesperson, having advised me against buying shoes which are 'grossly inappropriate' for my purposes, has no duty to refuse the sale if I insist on buying them. What are the implications of importing these consumer assumptions into the doctor–patient relationship? The most obvious implication is that medicine will cease to be a profession and will become a service industry. If that happens the ethics of medicine will completely change. Indeed, some might argue that the need for ethics of any kind will vanish because the discipline of the market will replace the need for ethics. But I prefer to say that traditional medical ethics (which have grown up to protect the vulnerable patient against exploitation) will be replaced by the ethics of consumerism—and this is certainly being encouraged by the government in the UK. Let us look briefly at the ethics of consumerism.

Consumer ethics tend to highlight the following concepts. Consumers must have *access* to the services or goods they require; they must have *choice* of the goods or services they require; and this will involve *competition* between suppliers and a fair balance in the market place between supplier and customer; consumers must have *adequate information* on the goods and services they require, and the information must be expressed in clear language; it must be possible for the customer to obtain *redress* in the event of poor services or goods; the products or services must be *safe and subject to regulation* to ensure safety.

Consumer ethics of this nature underlie the concept of the free market and it is certainly appropriate in some areas of life. The question is whether it is appropriate in health care. It has at least two important implications: health care becomes a commodity like any other in the market, and the carers comprise a service industry. It is not possible in this short introduction to discuss the far-reaching implications of such a change in ethos or to evaluate it. I shall simply note in summary that one and the same concept of patient autonomy is open to two different interpretations—and in the case of the second interpretation ('consumer autonomy') gives rise to a radically different view of medical practice from the traditional one. I am not here expressing a view as to whether this different view is better or worse than the traditional one in terms of health care delivery, but there is no doubt that there will be a basic change in the underlying ethic.

5. Utility and justice

Whether or not we adopt the traditional or the consumer view of the doctor–patient relationship we must come to terms with the need for rationing in health care. Some people may argue that rationing, although raising important issues, does not raise ethical issues. The assumption of this position is that ethics has to do only with the face-to-face situation. I believe this view to be inadequate. Questions of the supply and fair distribution of resources are matters of ethics, and the general ethical principles that are relevant are those of utility and justice. Utility is the principle concerned with maximizing outcomes or preferences. In older terminology it tells us to seek the greatest happiness of the greatest number. As such, the principle of utility says nothing about *how* the greatest happiness should be distributed; an aggregate of utility A might be greater than an aggregate of B, but we might still give our moral approval to the situation that produces B rather than A, on the grounds that in B the benefits are more fairly distributed. It has been a long-running debate within moral philosophy as to whether our moral judgement for B can still somehow be subsumed under the principle of utility. Without prejudging this debate it might be preferable to work with two principles rather than with the single principle of utility. We can then make explicit the moral tension between the claims of justice and fairness, or equality, on the one hand, and utility on the other. This question is of primary importance to the intensive care unit.

The ethical problems that derive from the tension between equality and utility arise in different areas of health care. One area is the distribution of health care. Granted standard services, how should they be distributed? If we emphasize the principle of utility then resources should be concentrated on large centres of population; but this is clearly unfair to those living in rural areas, who would be obliged to travel unreasonable distances for health care. There is the second question of *what* services should be available. Media attention, and indeed medical research interests, are typically directed towards the highly technical end of medicine, such as intensive care units, and because public imagination is captured by these services politicians are sympathetic towards the demands of prominent high-technology consultants. However, it is arguable whether this is the best use of scarce health care resources. Greater utility might result from putting the millions of pounds involved into health education, anti-smoking campaigns, and subsidies for fruit and vegetables in urban areas, than into heart transplant units.

There is a third area where there can be tensions between equality and utility and this is in the measurement of quality in health care (and indeed elsewhere, such as in the field of education). Utility commits us to evaluating outcomes, to setting targets, to auditing everything that can be audited, and many activities that cannot. Evaluation programmes, viewed in this way under the umbrella of 'utility', require the introduction of measurement scales, and if there are measurement scales there must be measurement units. The consequence of this is that what is not in measurable units tends to be regarded as unimportant. To put it differently, and controversially, quality is interpreted in quantitative terms, and consequently in some areas of health care, where quality is not easily quantifiable, quality is marginalized. For example, how is quality to be measured in the palliative area of health care? As a result of the desire to quantify (which is an implication of utility), there can be injustice in the evaluation of some services.

A fourth area where utility and equality can conflict is that of research. Medical research is important because it ensures continual improvement in the quality of patient care, and also the optimum use of scarce resources. Examples abound of such improvements—such as new laser techniques in surgery that are not only beneficial for patients but also good for scarce resources. Research is therefore an imperative of utility. However, randomized trials and other types of intervention involved in research may not be in the best interests of given patients (to say nothing of the animals also involved in the research). But codes of ethics always state that the interests of individual patients must be given priority over every other consideration. Some patients must therefore be treated unfairly in the interests of general utility. We could also describe this as a clash between beneficence or non-maleficence and utility. It is irrelevant to this conflict whether patients have consented or not (although, of course, their autonomy will also be infringed if they have not). This conflict seems irresolvable.

6. The virtues of compassion and self-development

I shall conclude with a discussion of two areas of health care ethics that have tended to be neglected, but are now being more stressed in nursing literature and indeed more generally in the feminist movement.

It has recently been argued that medical ethics stresses principles too much and feelings not enough—that caring, which is said to be a distinctively female virtue, has been neglected. I shall call this moral quality 'compassion', or suffering with someone.

The natural ingredients of compassion are part of the make-up of a normal human being. We all have the capacity to identify with others, to enter to some extent into their predicaments, and share their emotions. This capacity is displayed even in extreme situations, because it is the foundation of the strategy for dealing with terrorists who have taken hostages, (i.e. to delay doing anything as long as possible on the grounds that it is emotionally difficult to kill hostages if you have shared experiences with them). Compassion, however, is not just a matter of feeling with others—it is not passive. To have compassion is to be moved to *act*. (I prefer the old-fashioned term 'compassion' to the semi-technical term 'empathy' on the grounds that the latter suggests something passive.) All those in health care must attempt to develop in themselves the capacity for feeling with others; but compassion, like benevolence, requires an active response. In a similar way, the term 'sympathy' is ambiguous—being between passive and active modes of expression. If someone is described as 'very sympathetic' this might mean simply that he or she shared one's feelings, or that he or she went on to do something about one's predicament. To be compassionate, however, requires *both* responses.

There is also a cognitive side to compassion, which requires imaginative insight into a particular person's situation. This differs from a social science understanding of *types* of cases, such as 'the elderly patient'. To be an 'understanding person' is to have a biographer's or historian's flair for seeing just how this patient is where he or she is, *coupled with* compassion. Indeed, in health care the imaginative insight cannot exist without the compassion. Feeling and compassion provide us then with insight into the particular situation, as distinct from the typical case. Compassion cannot replace principles but provides an essential supplement to them.

The second neglected aspect of morality is the self-regarding aspect. Some philosophers deny that there can be a self-regarding side to morality, because they see morality as having an essentially social function, concerned only with regulating one's conduct *vis-à-vis* other members of society. Such a view has developed out of one strand in John Stuart Mill's thinking. Mill, in his essay *On liberty*, seems to be arguing that moral issues only arise when one's conduct harms other people. 'Yet, in the same work, Mill discusses 'self-development' (Chapter 3), where the importance of developing certain personality traits is stressed. As he puts it: 'It really is of importance not only what men do, but also what manner of men they are that do it'.[7] This view, that there are moral duties to cultivate in oneself certain characteristic human merits, goes back to Plato and Aristotle, and is taken up in a slightly different form by the Judaeo-Christian traditions. According to these traditions human nature can 'flourish' and should therefore be cultivated, or that we have a duty to cultivate the talents we have in trust. For Kant, the principle (or attitude) that is often stated in the form of: 'One ought to respect autonomous persons', really takes the form: 'Respect human nature, whether in your own person or in that of another'. In other words, Kant makes ample room for the idea of a self-regarding area of a morality.

Self-development is an important area of morality for those in the caring professions, and it is the more important in that its neglect can seem a virtue. It is quite common for professional carers to live a life of devotion to their patients, and as a result their own lives become empty and impoverished. They have cultivated their medical knowledge and skills only and have nothing else of themselves to give.

The duty of self-development can also be justified in terms of its benefits to other people. Since so much of the success of a doctor, nurse, dentist, or other health worker depends on the relationship each has with a patient, and since the nature of that relationship depends partly on the patient's perceptions of the helper, it is vital that the professional should be seen as an authentic human being who happens to be a doctor, nurse, or other carer. If a doctor is to give himself to others he must have something to give! There is a moral element in the most technical-seeming medical or nursing judgements. It is important, therefore, that these judgements should be the products not just of a technical, scientific mind, but of a humane and compassionate one. That is why it is important for the health care professional to be *more* than just that; to be a morally developed person who happens to follow a given professional path. Self-development, then, is good both for its own sake and for what it gives to patients, friends, and families.

7. Conclusion

In this chapter I have identified some of the main principles and concepts that are essential to discussions of medical ethics. I have also stressed that our interpretation of these principles is influenced by the ethos (or culture) of the health care professions, and more widely by changing social attitudes and economic necessities. The history of medical ethics can be seen as the evolution of the doctor–patient relationship; but more recent social and economic changes are likely to have a radical effect on the traditional relationship and may change it from a professional relationship into a consumer relationship.

Notes

1. Jonsen, A.R. (1990). *The new medicine and the old ethics*. Harvard University Press, Cambridge, MA.
2. Percival, T. (1803). *Medical ethics*, (ed. Chauncey Leake (1976)), p. 71. Krieger, New York.
3. Paris, J.J. *et al.* (1993). Sounding board. *New England Journal of Medicine*, **329**, 354–7.
4. Veatch, R.M. and Spicer, C.M. (1992). Medically futile care; the role of the physician in setting limits. *American Journal of Law and Medicine*, **18**, 15–36.
5. *Re J (a minor)* Court of Appeal (10 June 1992). Lord Chief Justice Donaldson. For discussion, see Kerreth, R. (1992). British judges cannot order doctors to treat. *Hastings Centre Report*, **22**, 3–4.
6. Mill, John Stuart (1859). *On liberty*, (ed. Mary Warnock (1962)). Collins, London.
7. Note 6, p. 188.

Brain Death and the Persistent Vegetative State

Bryan Jennett

The life-saving and life-sustaining technologies of intensive care developed in the late 1950s made it possible for patients who had suffered severe brain damage to survive, at least for a time. Previously, most such injuries would have proved fatal. Doctors were then presented with the problem, largely of their own making, of some patients so severely brain damaged that survival was judged as being of no benefit to them. The question then arose of the doctor's duty to preserve and prolong life in such circumstances. This was a situation where the traditional ethical framework of medicine provided no adequate guidance, and which also presented legal problems. However, the last 25 years has seen medicine, moral philosophy and the law debating these issues at length and they are now largely resolved, at least in regard to brain death.

Patients with irrecoverable severe brain damage may be brain dead or be in a persistent vegetative state (PVS). In the former it is the brainstem that is irreversibly out of action, in the latter the cerebral cortex. These result in two contrasting physiological situations and two quite different problems for decision-making. In brain death, the paradox is a patient whose brain is no longer functioning but whose heart continues to beat. In the vegetative state, the paradox is of a patient who is awake but not aware. Even with maximal support the ventilator-dependent brain-dead patient will maintain a beating heart usually for only a week or two, whereas the spontaneously breathing vegetative patient treated with tube feeding and basic nursing care may survive for years. A decision to withdraw life-sustaining technology from a brain-dead patient therefore brings final cardiac arrest forward by only a few days, whereas death is not imminent for the stable vegetative patient. As these situations are so different they are best dealt with separately.

1. Brain death

It was inevitable that the increasing availability of mechanical ventilation and the development of cardiopulmonary resuscitation as a routine in the 1950s would lead to some rescued patients being left with a beating heart after the brain was dead. The first report of this was in 1959 from Paris where Mollaret and Goulon termed this state 'coma dépassé'[1] Ten years later the Ad Hoc Committee of the Harvard Medical School published criteria for its diagnosis,[2] as a basis for discontinuing ventilation.

Essential to the concept of brain death is the recognition that death is a process rather than an event. Various organs and tissues cease to function, and later necrose, at different stages in the process of death, and when death is declared it is to some extent arbitrary. The World Medical Association Declaration of Sydney in 1968 proposed that death is when the body as an integrated whole has irreversibly ceased to function, rather than when all organs and tissues are dead. From biblical times the cessation of breathing was the usual sign of death, but its unreliability caused concern about premature diagnosis. In 1740, a paper declared that the only certain sign of death was putrefaction, and at that time there were devices that enabled those prematurely consigned to mortuaries to signal that they were still alive, by means of strings going up from the fingers to a pulley and a bell. The invention of the stethoscope in the early 1800s focused attention on the heartbeat as the ultimate sign of life, and now we have brainstem function as yet another.

There are three common sequences that lead to death. Most often, cardiac arrest is the initial event and soon the cerebral cortex ceases to function; later the brainstem also fails: and then respiration stops. Less often, respiratory arrest begins the sequence, leading to anoxia of the cortex, and then brainstem failure, whilst cardiac arrest may not occur for 15 to 30 minutes. Sometimes, the brainstem fails first, followed by respiratory arrest, with anoxic cardiac arrest occurring later. If artificial ventilation restores oxygenation after the brainstem is dead but before the heart stops then ultimate cardiac arrest may be delayed for many days. It is, however, a mistake to consider that there are two kinds of death—that evidenced by cardiorespiratory arrest, and that by lack of brainstem function. This is because cardiorespiratory arrest is considered to indicate death only when it has lasted long enough to produce brainstem death. When patients are successfully resuscitated from cardiac arrest or have been subjected to therapeutically controlled stoppage of the heart during surgery, we do not claim that they had been dead. It is, therefore, brainstem death that is the central feature of all sequences of death, whereas the state of continued cardiac function after this has occurred is an artefact of nature resulting from technological intervention.

A distinction is sometimes drawn between brainstem death and whole-brain death. However, the function of the cerebral cortex is dependent on upward impulses from the reticular formation in the brainstem, and therefore when the brainstem is dead the brain as a whole cannot function. This is not to deny that some cells in the cerebral cortex and basal ganglia may continue to survive for a time, but they are not able to maintain the function of the brain as a whole. The logic of the situation is therefore that if the brainstem is dead the whole brain is dead. It is also now accepted that if the whole brain is dead the person is dead. This last concept is explicitly stated in the UK Royal Colleges memorandum of 1979,[4] which states that the time of death is when brainstem death is confirmed and not some later time when the heart stops. This is important to explain to those involved in procedures associated with organ donation, when there may be a delay of several hours before the ventilator is withdrawn and the heart stops. It is easy to refer carelessly to withdrawing life support or letting the patient die, when in fact ventilation is being stopped in a patient who is already dead. No legislation has been deemed necessary in this country to acknowledge this additional means of diagnosing death. However, in 1970, the State of Kansas was the first of many US states to bring in a brain death law, and Finland led the Europeans a year later. Most of these laws recognize only that death can be declared by neurological criteria—they do not specify what these should be. This is a matter for clinical guidelines and there is some variation in these from one country to another, and in the US between one hospital and another.

2. Diagnosis of brain death: UK criteria

These criteria were published by the UK Royal Colleges in 1976[3] and a further memorandum in 1979[4] confirmed these and indicated that death could be declared once the criteria were satisfied. A feature of the diagnostic criteria is the emphasis on satisfying the preconditions before considering the tests to confirm that the brainstem is dead. There are four preconditions. The patient:

(1) *must* be in deep coma;

(2) *must* be apnoeic (and therefore on a ventilator);

(3) *must* have irrecoverable structural brain damage;

(4) and reversible causes of brainstem depression *must* have been excluded.

Common causes of brain damage leading to brain death are severe head injury and spontaneous intracranial haemorrhage, but a few result from brain tumour or intracranial infection. Some cases follow delayed resuscitation after cardiac arrest from various causes including anoxia and drug overdose. Reversible causes of brainstem depression include depressant drugs, neuromuscular blocking agents used for intubation during resuscitations or as an adjunct to mechanical ventilation, hypothermia, and gross metabolic abnormalities. These various factors may not be the sole cause of brainstem depression but can aggravate the effect of structural lesions. Screening for drugs will not normally be necessary when there is a clear-cut story of sudden coma from injury. As for establishing the irrecoverability of the brain damage, enough time should elapse to correct temporary causes of brainstem depression such as hypotension, hypoxia, and raised intracranial pressure. Normally, the diagnosis would not be considered in less than 6 hours but when the cause is anoxic damage or when drugs are suspected the diagnosis should be delayed for at least 24 hours.

The tests to confirm that there is no residual brainstem function are simple to perform and interpret:

- there should be no pupillary or corneal reflexes;

- there should be no movement of the facial muscles to pain, or of the throat muscles to movement of the endotracheal tube;

- the caloric vestibulo-ocular reflex should be absent (no eye movements following irrigation of the external auditory meatus with at least 20 ml of ice cold water on each side).

Only when these reflexes are all found to be absent is the final *crucial test* applied, to confirm apnoea:

- there should be no respiratory movements when disconnection of the ventilator allows the $P\text{CO}_2$ to rise.

The UK criteria required $P\text{CO}_2$ to reach 50 mmHg (6.65 kPa) but US codes recommend 60 mmHg (8.0 kPa). The rate of rise of $P\text{CO}_2$ in brain-dead patients can be slow,[5] and to attain this level in 10 minutes requires that the $P\text{CO}_2$ be greater than 40 mmHg (5.3 kPa) before disconnection. This can be achieved by reducing the tidal volume or by ventilating with 95 per cent oxygen and 5 per cent carbon dioxide for 5 minutes. To ensure that damaging hypoxia does not occur during disconnection pre-oxygenation with 100 per cent oxygen for 10 minutes before disconnection is recommended and the maintenance during disconnection of 6 litres per minute of oxygen delivered down a catheter in the trachea. Advice from experts is required for patients with pre-existing chronic respiratory insufficiency who normally depend on an hypoxic drive for respiration and may be unresponsive to raised $P\text{CO}_2$.

The UK criteria specify that two doctors, not members of the transplant team, should be involved in testing, one of them a consultant and the other a senior registrar or consultant. They may examine the patient separately or together, and they should each repeat the tests on a second occasion. Provided the preconditions have been met before the first tests the interval between the two assessments need be no more than 30 minutes. Note that these criteria require no confirmatory laboratory tests.

The 1968 Harvard criteria recommended demonstrating absence of cerebral activity on electroencephalography (EEG), but this was declared optional by that institution a year later.[6] EEG is still frequently used in the US and in other countries, and sometimes in the UK. In practice, it is less useful than might be expected, partly because it reflects activity in the cerebral hemispheres rather than the brainstem (and some residual activity may persist after unequivocal brainstem death), and because securing an isoelectric EEG recording can be technically difficult in the electronically active environment of an intensive care unit. Those who use it sometimes say that they do so to convince the family rather than to make a diagnosis. Another possible confirmatory test is to demonstrate absence of cerebral circulation over a period of time, either visually by angiography or by showing no entry of radioactive agents injected systemically. Both require technical equipment and expertise and neither is wholly reliable; they are virtually never used in the UK and rarely in the US.

Definitive guidance on the diagnosis of brain death in children has been given by a US Task Force.[7] In the UK the British Paediatric Association has suggested that over the age of 2 months the adult criteria can be used, but that data for younger children are insufficient to define guidelines.[8]

3. Validity of the criteria

These criteria have now been applied to many thousands of patients, many of whom were ventilated until cardiac asystole before clinicians gained the confidence to discontinue ventilation once brain death had been diagnosed. Not one case is on record as having recovered after the UK criteria were satisfied, according to Pallis (1990) who listed over 1900 published cases.[9] None the less, sporadic press reports of patients allegedly recovering after supposedly having been brain dead appeared during the 1970s and these culminated in a challenge on BBC TV in 1980 about whether organ donors were in fact always definitely dead before organs were removed. The critics were mostly from other countries (particularly the US) who seemed mainly concerned that the UK criteria did not require an EEG. The final conclusion was that the original criteria did not need to be modified,[10] whereas subsequent guidelines in the US stressed that the use of EEG was still optional.[11]

However, it is prudent to be alert to the misunderstandings that can arise in this sensitive area of medicine. Most centre on the issue of organ donation and the suspicion that eagerness to secure organs might tempt doctors to make a premature diagnosis of brain death. An allegation may be made that a patient recovered after 'they nearly removed his kidneys'. A likely explanation is that the family was told soon after an acute episode of brain damage that the outlook was almost hopeless, but that the results of resuscitation were still awaited. Today when such a prognosis is given, families themselves sometimes raise the possibility of organ donation. The response to this should be to indicate that it is too soon to be sure that there will be no recovery (and certainly too soon to diagnose brain death). However, doctors may be tempted to accept this offer even though noting that diagnostic tests will be needed later. As such patients occasionally do recover, or at least survive for a time, it is easy to see how in retrospect it may seem as though organs were nearly taken. The same may happen when a reversible cause of brainstem depression such as drug overdose is discovered. Clearly these are not examples of recovery after the formal diagnosis of brain death. Misunderstandings can also arise in the intensive care unit when bystanders observe the activity of spinal reflexes in patients declared brain dead. In fact, these become more active the longer ventilation is continued after brain death, and they may be precipitated by the removal of organs.

The best safeguard against such serious allegations is never to consider the diagnosis of brain death until the preconditions have been met, to use widely accepted diagnostic criteria, to have two doctors involved, and always to allow enough time to be certain that the situation is not reversible. These conditions have been established in the UK by the Health Department's Code of Practice published in 1979, and revised in 1983,[12] which reproduces the UK Colleges' criteria and memoranda, as well as giving detailed guidelines for the removal of organs for transplantation. This has been widely distributed and the diagnostic criteria have recently been reproduced yet again in the form of a check-list for inclusion in the patient's notes.[13] In practice, there now seems little continuing controversy in the UK about brain death, a concept that both the public at large and the families actually involved seem able to accept.

4. Procedure in other countries

The guidelines produced by a group of US medical consultants[11] for the President's Commission on defining death in 1981 appear not to have been widely accepted,[14] let alone adopted, according to surveys of neurosurgeons and neurologists.[15,16] Indeed, most of the 106 responders in the first survey did not favour national guidelines and in fact they used widely varying criteria. Not only did 16 per cent not test for apnoea at all, but only 20 per cent used rigorous apnoea testing as specified in the UK criteria. Although the 1981 guidelines declared that EEG was an optional test, two-thirds of the 1984 survey still used this test, 36 per cent requiring two flat EEGs, and 29 per cent only one. Only 6 per cent used angiography to establish absent cerebral circulation. Another survey[17] revealed that a considerable minority of 195 doctors and nurses were confused about the difference between brain death and the vegetative state—many believing that the latter could also justify declaring a patient dead. This led to an editorial surprisingly entitled 'Appropriate confusion over "brain death" '.[18]

There is no authoritative review of the current situation in European countries, a number of which have followed the US by enacting legislation. Italy alone has laws that actually specify the diagnostic criteria to be used, rather than the requirement that brain death be diagnosed 'by currently accepted criteria'. A number of European countries still use EEG and some require angiographic evidence of absent cerebral circulation—some of them doing so only when organ donation is envisaged. It has always seemed illogical to have different criteria for death when transplantation is on the agenda. In the UK, it has always been emphasized that both the diagnosis of brain death and subsequent discontinuation of ventilation are part of normal good practice, regardless of organ donation.

Some other countries have held out against the recognition of brain death, although some have recently yielded to some extent, according to Pallis.[9] In India a code very similar to that of the UK has emerged, whilst organ donation from heart-beating donors has been declared permissible by religious authorities in Saudi Arabia. In Israel, the Ministry of Health has approved brain death and some transplants have proceeded although discussion in parliament has been avoided as too sensitive in the light of orthodox Jewish teaching. Japan has still to approve the concept although it is addressing the issue through the Ministry of Health. Denmark remains the only developed country to have actually rejected brain death through its National Council of Ethics (of which only 3 of 17 members are doctors).[19] It nonetheless accepts that brain death indicates that the death process has begun and is irreversible, and it permits removal of organs while the heart is still beating, which is considered to end the death process but not to be the cause of death. This has been described as 'wanting it both ways' by Lamb in one of a series of commentaries on this decision.[20]

5. Frequency of brain death and organ donation

Although it has been emphasized that brain death is a phenomenon that developed without any relationship to transplantation, it is inevitable that research into the frequency of brain death has stemmed from attempts to estimate the potential pool of organ donors. In 1981 Jennett and Hessett analysed 1228 kidney donors, to find that most came from general intensive care units (ICUs) and that many of these units were in District general hospitals rather than teaching hospitals.[21] This emphasized the need for criteria that could be used by a wide range of different specialists. About half the donors had suffered head injury and almost a third intracranial haemorrhage. By extrapolation from data about head injury epidemiology and its contribution to brain death it was estimated that there might be as many as 4000 cases of brain death each year in UK. A more recent prospective study of English and Welsh ICUs has led to a lower estimate of incidence—only half this number of potentially brain dead and a third of confirmed cases.[22-24] Both this national survey and a study in one regional neurosurgical unit[25] showed that a quarter of possibly brain dead patients were never tested for brain death, although all but 6 per cent of relatives were asked about donation, of whom 30 per cent refused to consent. About a fifth of those tested were medically unsuitable for organ donation. As a consequence of these various factors only a third of the possibly brain dead and a half of those confirmed actually became donors. The code of practice published by the Health Departments makes it clear that there is no legal objection to the administration of drugs (including intravenous fluids) to maintain the condition of organs once brain death has been diagnosed, but that only very occasionally is it justified to initiate ventilation before death with the purpose of preserving organ function rather than to improve the chances of recovery of the patient. However, recent studies indicate that a considerable number of patients presently die outside ICUs from cerebrovascular accidents (stroke) so severe that artificial ventilation is not instituted, but that if such patients were electively ventilated there could be a marked increase in the number of organs available for transplantation.[26,27] Such practice has been developed in at least one hospital, where it was considered to be ethically acceptable and was supported by the families of affected patients.[26] However, there is some controversy about the legal, ethical, and resource implications of such a procedure, which would involve treating patients who were not yet dead by methods not designed to benefit them, and using ICU resources for the sole purpose of providing organs for transplantation (see Chapter 10).

6. The persistent vegetative state (PVS)

This is a clinical syndrome resulting from a wide range of acute and chronic conditions, with greatly differing pathologies, that leave a patient with no evidence of function in the cerebral cortex. However, because the brainstem is relatively intact, including the arousal mechanisms, these patients are awake with long periods of spontaneous eye opening. After head injury, the eyes normally open after 2 to 4 weeks, but with non-traumatic coma, which is not associated with any concussion of the brainstem, patients may become vegetative within a few days, even within 24 hours, of the ictus (brain insult). There is, however, no evidence of awareness—no sustained, reproducible, purposeful or voluntary response, no commands obeyed, and not even a single word spoken. Yet a wide but variable range of reflex activities can persist, including blinking to visual threat, unsustained visual tracking of moving objects, withdrawal of spastic limbs from a painful stimulus which may cause an increase in pulse and respiration rates and in blood pressure, perhaps a grimace and a groan. But these responses do not imply that there is any experience of pain or suffering. Reflex swallowing and vestibulo-ocular reflexes usually persist, and some emotional behaviour commonly occurs—brief smiling, weeping, or even laughter, but unrelated to meaningful stimuli.

No reliable laboratory tests are available to confirm that a patient is vegetative. Computed tomography (CT) scanning shows marked brain atrophy, but similar degrees have been reported from age-matched controls with severe dementia who retain some conscious behaviour. However, the absence of atrophy some months after an acute episode of brain damage could indicate that some degree of recovery from the vegetative state might occur, and this was indeed a feature of two widely reported cases. EEG recordings are very variable, most patients showing delta or theta activity, but 25 per cent have a near normal alpha rhythm. However, such EEG activity is usually unresponsive to external stimuli. Some 5 per cent have an isoelectric EEG record. Cortical evoked responses to somatosensory stimuli are often absent, but may persist in PVS patients, whereas a number of patients with absent responses regain some consciousness. Some patients regain consciousness although the EEG is getting worse, whereas others have an improving EEG without clinical recovery. The most promising investigation is positron emission tomography (PET), although presently it is available only for research purposes. One study showed PVS patients to have a cerebral metabolic rate for glucose less than 50 per cent of normal in the cortex and basal ganglia, a level only previously recorded in deep barbiturate coma[28]. However, another study[29] also examined severely brain-damaged patients with some residual consciousness, and one such patient had a lower metabolic rate than the highest level found in the group of PVS patients—so perhaps even this is not a wholly reliable test. The diagnosis of this behavioural state is therefore essentially clinical, depending on evidence from skilled observers over a period of time.

When Plum and the present author described and named this syndrome we referred only to its resulting from an acute brain insult.[30] It is now recognized that there may be as many cases resulting from progressive dementia, such as Alzheimer's disease, and in children from metabolic and developmental brain disorders. The acute cases may be traumatic or non-traumatic. About 10 to 14 per cent of patients admitted with a severe head injury are vegetative a month later, which is about 20 per cent of survivors. In a series of 500 cases of non-traumatic coma, 39 per cent survived for a month and 30 per cent of these were vegetative.[31] Hypoxia accounted for 70 per cent of which 70 per cent had had a cardiac arrest, the rest profound hypotension or various kinds of asphyxiation including strangulation and drowning. Other non-traumatic causes are strokes of various kinds, hypoglycaemia, and intracranial tumours or infections. Surveys in Japan and The Netherlands of patients vegetative 3 to 6 months after acute insults found that 40 per cent were traumatic but a recent American aggregate of published cases, at least 1 month after an acute incident showed 70 per cent to be traumatic.[32] This high percentage may reflect the number of head injury reports from neurosurgeons in the literature, rather than the true frequency.

Pathological findings vary with the cause. Following hypoxia or hypoglycaemia there is widespread necrosis of neurones in the cortex and basal ganglia. After head injury the main lesion is extensive tearing of subcortical white matter, the diffuse axonal injury that results from shearing injury at the moment of impact. A relatively undamaged cortex is then effectively isolated, as evidenced by the completeness of late degeneration in the corticospinal tract. Traumatic cases often have additional extensive ischaemic brain damage in the cortex and basal ganglia. The extent and distribution of the brain damage varies considerably from case to case and this doubtless accounts for the variations in the reflex responsiveness of different patients; moreover, there is overlap with the findings in very severely brain-damaged patients who have some residual consciousness. There is therefore no single lesion that always produces the vegetative state—rather it occurs when there is no longer the critical amount of cerebral cortex, surviving and connected, that is required for consciousness.

How many PVS patients there are in the community is uncertain, with surveys from different countries producing varying estimates. This partly reflects whether cases are sought in all of the many places that PVS patients may be—in acute hospitals, nursing homes, and even at home; whereas some surveys are limited to acute cases, and others to adults or children. Another variable is how long patients need to be vegetative before being counted as in PVS. Recent American consensus statements propose that being vegetative one month *after* an acute insult[33] or *for* one month are sufficient to define PVS. However, Japanese surveys were limited to those vegetative at three months and in the Netherlands six months was required. These variations affect not only estimates of the number of PVS patients, but also statements about prognosis, because many of those vegetative at 1 month either die or recover consciousness during the next 3 to 12 months. Thus in the UK, there are probably some 1200 newly vegetative patients each year 1 month after an acute incident, but only 250 of these would be alive and vegetative after 6 months. An estimate of 1000–1500 cases vegetative for at least 1 month in the UK, from acute and chronic causes, would approximate to estimates in Japan and France. In the US, estimates are 3 to 5 times higher, perhaps due to the greater frequency of severe head injuries, to more attention being given to ascertaining cases from chronic conditions and in children, and also to more vigorous rescue and support of severely brain-damaged patients.

In deciding the appropriate management of PVS patients the most important consideration is the remaining potential for recovery. A number of patients who are vegetative for a time after an acute insult do regain consciousness. However, a distinction should be made between recovery of some limited degree of consciousness and the restoration of useful function. Most patients who recover after being vegetative for several months never speak or are capable of only occasional monosyllabic utterances or of obeying occasional commands; they do not become fully interactive persons with a quality of life that can be enjoyed even at a limited level. Some, however, do regain a degree of independence—although how this term is defined is important. According to the Glasgow Outcome Scale,[34] which is widely used for assessing outcome after acute brain damage, independence indicates the patient's capacity to organize his or her own life on a day-to-day basis without the support or prompting of family or carers. A more limited degree of independence applies only to activities of daily life—which usually means the capacity for self-care within the sick room but requiring the intervention of others every day for some activities. In the following data about recovery, 'independence' refers to the higher level of social independence, defined above according to the Glasgow Scale.

The most important factor determining potential for recovery is the duration of the vegetative state. Other factors are the cause of brain damage (traumatic cases recover better) and the patient's age (children do better). The probability of recovery of consciousness and of independence has been analysed by the US Multi-Society Task Force for an aggregate of 754 patients whose outcomes have been published in medical journals.[32] Of patients vegetative one month after an acute insult, regardless of age and diagnosis, 34 per cent were dead by the end of a year, 24 per cent were still vegetative, and 43 per cent had regained consciousness with 18 per cent becoming independent. Of non-traumatic cases, however, only 14 per cent regained consciousness and 2 per cent became independent. After three months the chances even of regaining consciousness after non-traumatic damage was only 7 per cent and 3 per cent for adults and children, respectively, and only one such patient became independent after being three months in a vegetative state. After six months only a few children with head injury ever regained independence. Exceptional cases of late recovery are reported from time to time, often in the non-medical press, with inadequate details to substantiate the claims. Only five such cases were accepted by the US Task Force as valid, and all were left very severely disabled without independence.

A number of authoritative bodies have now made recommendations about when the possibility of recovery from the vegetative state can no longer be considered a reasonable prospect. Although some consider that 1–3 months is long enough after anoxic brain damage all require 6–12 months after trauma. In 1990, the American Medical Association suggested 3 months after anoxic damage, 12 months after trauma, but only 6 months in head-injured patients over 50 years of age.[35] At that time the various late recoveries mentioned above had already all been published and it was estimated that the error rate in applying these recommendations would be less than one in a thousand. In 1993, the British Medical Association accepted the more conservative 12 months for all patients.[36] The most recent American recommendation (1994), based on a review of published cases, is 3 months for non-traumatic and 12 months for traumatic cases.[32]

Another aspect of prognosis is how long PVS patients survive. The average survival is 3–4 years but several cases have been recorded living for 10–20 years, one for 37 years, and another for 40 years. Once the patient has survived the first year there is a greater chance of prolonged survival. Eventually death is usually due to pulmonary or urinary tract infection, and when this occurs may depend on how vigorously such complications are treated.

All are agreed that a high standard of supportive nursing care, adequate nutrition, and physiotherapy are important in the early months in order to provide the best chance of spontaneous recovery. However, the conclusion of the US Task Force in 1994 was that no treatment actually promotes recovery from the vegetative state.[32] None of the unexpected late recoveries reported in the literature appear to have resulted from a particular treatment regime.

Given these medical facts, the ethical issue is whether, once there is considered no likelihood of useful recovery, doctors are obliged to prolong life by continuing tube feeding and the treatment of complications. The crucial question is whether such prolongation of life can be considered a benefit to the patient, and who is to decide this. Some have described vegetative survival as a fate worse than death, and some ethicists consider that such patients have lost person-hood, therefore defining them as non-dead non-persons. Questionnaires about advance directives for life-sustaining treatment indicate that the vast majority of responders do not want any life-saving or life-sustaining treatment if they are in a vegetative state with no prospect of reasonable recovery.[37,38] That prolonging life in the vegetative state is of no benefit is a view already taken by many courts in the US and by all nine judges in the Bland case in the UK,[39] (Mr Anthony Bland was a 17-year-old victim of the Hillsborongh football stadium disaster in April 1989. He suffered brain damage and existed in a PVS state from then until 1993.) Several cases since Bland have been decided similarly in the English High Court. Most public comment in the US and UK has supported these legal decisions. Several religious authorities in different denominations have also indicated that a life devoid of almost all the attributes of a human being is one that there is no moral obligation to save or prolong. However, there is a minority of vitalists who maintain that the preservation of life of whatever kind is in itself good and that to deny this is to challenge the sanctity of life. But all the judges in the Bland case specifically referred to the fact that this was not a principle that should always take precedence over other considerations. The relatives of PVS patients form another constituency to consider. A study of 33 relatives of mainly elderly PVS patients in US nursing homes found less than one in five willing to consider withdrawal of life-sustaining treatment, and that two-thirds wanted active intervention to reduce the risk to life posed by a new medical complication.[40]

The view that has emerged from the majority of medical, ethical, and legal pronouncements about the management of permanently vegetative patients is that withdrawal of life-sustaining nutrition and hydration is an acceptable course of action.[35,36,41,42] This is seen as a logical extension of the now widely accepted practice of withholding or withdrawing life-saving or life-sustaining treatment when this is considered to be of no benefit to the patient, or when only limited benefit is outweighed by the burdens that such treatment imposes (see Chapter 4). Such treatment is considered not to be in the patient's best interest, and there is, therefore, no moral or legal obligation to provide this treatment. However, whereas most other decisions to limit treatment are made for patients whose death is imminent, and when one reason for limiting treatment is to avoid prolonging the suffering of a dying patient, the PVS patient does not face imminent death and by definition is not suffering. None the less, he or she can be considered to have had tube feeding initiated as a trial of treatment, in the hope that recovery might occur; once a year has passed without any sign of recovery that trial of treatment can be considered to have failed. In acute crises treatment withdrawal is usually considered after a trial of treatment that has lasted only hours or days, whereas in PVS patients it has lasted much longer. Another aspect is the question of resources, and whether prolonging the life of a PVS patient can be justified when these are restricted, remembering that justice in the distribution of health care resources is the fourth principle of medical ethics.[43, 44]

Some have argued that nutrition and hydration do not constitute medical treatment that could be withdrawn, but are part of basic care owed to every person under all circumstances. This view has been rejected by a range of bodies that have made declarations about the vegetative state, including medical, ethical, and legal authorities. Their view is that it is substituting a lost physiological function (efficient swallowing) just as ventilation or dialysis substitute for lack of respiratory or renal function. The symbolic significance of assuaging the thirst and hunger of another person by attending to these needs is thought not to apply to the tube feeding of an insentient PVS patient. Yet another concern is whether death after withdrawal of tube feeding is unpleasant to witness—accepting that it can cause no suffering to the patient. The evidence is that electrolyte imbalance and renal failure soon produces coma, and compassionate nursing assures a peaceful and dignified death.[45]

It now remains to consider who should make the decision that treatment should be withdrawn. Many are agreed that if the patient has made an advance directive (living will) indicating clearly that he or she did not wish for life-prolonging treatment if vegetative, then that wish should be honoured (see Chapter 5). The cause of death would then be considered to be underlying brain damage, not the withdrawal of treatment. There would therefore seem little danger of doctors being accused of murder, assisting suicide, or euthanasia—as many US judges and all nine judges in the UK Tony Bland case have emphasized. But such directives are the exception, particularly in younger patients who are frequent victims of acute episodes of brain damage. The doctor has then to decide what is in the patient's best interests, on the basis of weighing the balance between the benefits and burdens of alternative treatments—whether or not to use antibiotics to counter infective complications, or to continue or withdraw tube feeding. Such a decision should be made only after full consultation with and the agreement of the family. They are usually judged to be in the best position to know what this patient would want done, given his or her values and any opinions that he or she might have expressed informally about his or her treatment if in such a state.

Although the decision to withdraw treatment from a PVS patient may seem no different from other treatment-limiting decisions that are made daily in hospital, for the various reasons already outlined there is often a wish to formalize this particular decision. The US courts have decided many such cases, usually because hospital attorneys have refused to allow their doctors to act in what they agree to be in their patient's best interests, for fear of litigation.[46] However, many judges in the US now advise that it is not appropriate for such cases to come to court, but that doctors and families should reach this decision between themselves. Courts would be required only when there are no family members to act as surrogates or proxy decision-makers, or if there is some dispute between the parties involved. However, the judges in the Tony Bland case recommended that future cases in the UK should each come for judicial review—although some hinted that this might be a temporary arrangement and that once more experience was gained a more informal approach might be agreed. Indeed the Law Commission[47] and the Scottish Law Commission[48] have each suggested means by which applications to a court could be dispensed with. By contrast the House of Lords Select Committee,[49] set up after the Tony Bland case, has recently recommended that a new kind of judicial forum be established to consider decisions about special categories of treatment for incompetent patients. This would seem to apply to decisions about withholding tube feeding from PVS patients. The Committee was unable to decide whether tube feeding should be considered as medical treatment that could be withdrawn—but considered that withdrawal should seldom be required if a policy of withholding antibiotics was instituted at an earlier stage. Experience, however, teaches that prolonged survival is not uncommon even when infections are not treated.

Notes

1. Mollaret, P. and Goulon, M. (1959). Le coma dépassé. *Revue Neurologic,* **101**, 3–15.
2. Ad Hoc Committee of the Harvard Medical School (1968). Report on examining the definition of brain death. *Journal of the American Medical Association,* **205**, 85–8.
3. Conference of Medical Royal Colleges and their Faculties in the UK (1976). *British Medical Journal,* **2**, 1187–8.
4. Conference of Medical Royal Colleges and their Faculties in the UK (1979). Diagnosis of death. *British Medical Journal,* **1**, 322.
5. Benzel, E.C., *et al.* (1979). The apnoea test for the determination of brain death. *Journal of Neurosurgery,* **71**, 191–4.
6. Beecher, H.K. (1968). After the 'definition of irreversible coma'. *New England Journal of Medicine,* **281**, 1070–1.
7. Task Force for the Determination of Brain Death in Children (1987). Guidelines for the determination of brain death in children. *Archives of Neurology,* **44**, 587–8.
8. British Paediatric Association (1991). Working Party Report: *Diagnosis of brain stem death in infants and children.* British Paediatric Association, London.
9. Pallis, C. (1990). Brain stem death. In *Head injury,* (ed. R. Braakman), *Handbook of clinical neurology,* Vol. 57. Elsevier, Amsterdam.
10. Robson, J.G. (1981). Brain death. *British Medical Journal,* **283**, 505.
11. President's Commission (1981). Guidelines for the determination of death. *Journal of the American Medical Association,* **246**, 2184–6.
12. Health Departments of Great Britain and Northern Ireland (1983). *Cadaveric organs for transplantation: a code of practice including the diagnosis of brain death.* HMSO, London.

13. O'Brien M.D. (1990). Criteria for diagnosing brain stem death. *British Medical Journal*, 301, 108–9.
14. President's Commission (1981). *Defining death. Medical, legal and ethical issues in the determination of death*. US Government Printing Office, Washington, DC.
15. Black, P. McL. and Zervas, N.T. (1984). Declaration of brain death in neurosurgical and neurological practice. *Neurosurgery*, 15, 170–4.
16. Earnest, M.P., Beresford, R, and McIntyre, H.B. (1986). Testing for apnoea in suspected brain death: methods used by 129 clinicians. *Neurology*, 36, 42–4.
17. Youngner, S.J., *et al.* (1989). 'Brain death' and organ retrieval: a cross-sectional survey acknowledging concepts among health professionals. *Journal of the American Medical Association*, 261, 2205–10.
18. Wikler, D. and Weisbard, A.J. (1989). Appropriate confusion over 'brain death'. *Journal of the American Medical Association*, 261, 2246.
19. Rix, B.A. (1990). Danish Ethics Council rejects brain death as the criterion of death. *Journal of Medical Ethics*, 16, 5–7.
20. Lamb, D. (1990). Wanting it both ways. *Journal of Medical Ethics*, 16, 8–9.
21. Jennett, B. and Hessett, C. (1981). Brain death in Britain as reflected in renal donors. *British Medical Journal*, 283, 359–68.
22. Gore, S.M., Hindes, C.J., and Rutherford, A.J. (1989). Organ donation from intensive care units in England. *British Medical Journal*, 299, 1193–7.
23. Gore, S.M., Taylor, R.M.R., and Wallwork, J. (1991). Availability of transplantable organs from brain stem dead donors in intensive care units. *British Medical Journal*, 302, 149–53.
24. Gore, S.M., Cable, D.J., and Holland, A.J. (1992). Organ donation from intensive care units in England and Wales: two year confidential audit of deaths in intensive care. *British Medical Journal*, 204, 349–55.
25. Gentleman, D., Easton, J., and Jennett, B. (1990). Brain death and organ donation in a neurosurgical unit: an audit of recent practice. *British Medical Journal*, 301, 1203–6.
26. Feest, T.G., *et al.* (1990). Protocol for increasing organ donation after cerebrovascular deaths in a district general hospital. *Lancet*, 335, 1133–5.
27. Salih, M.A.M., *et al.* (1991). Potential availability of cadaver organs for transplantation. *British Medical Journal*, 302, 1053–5.
28. Levy, D.E., *et al.* (1987). Differences in cerebral blood flow and glucose utilisation in vegetative versus locked-in patients. *Annals of Neurology*, 22, 673–82.
29. De Volder, A.G., *et al.* (1990). Brain glucose metabolism in post-anoxic syndrome. Positron emission tomographic study. *Archives of Neurology*, 47, 197–204.
30. Jennett, B. and Plum F. (1972). Persistent vegetative state after brain damage. A syndrome in search of a name. *Lancet*, 1, 734–7.
31. Levy, D.E., *et al.* (1981). Prognosis in non-traumatic coma. *Annals of Internal Medicine*, 94, 293–301.
32. Multi-Society Task Force (1995). Statement on medical aspects of the persistent vegetative state. *New England Journal of Medicine*, 330, 1499–1508, 1572–9.
33. American Neurological Association Committee on Ethical Affairs (1993). Persistent vegetative state. *Annals of Neurology*, 33, 286–90.
34. Jennett, B. and Bond, M.R. (1975). Assessment of outcome after severe brain damage. *Lancet*, 1, 480–4.
35. American Medical Association Council on Ethical and Judicial Affairs (1990).

Persistent vegetative state and the decision to withdraw or withhold life support. *Journal of the American Medical Association*, **263**, 426–30.

36. BMA (British Medical Association) (1993). Guidelines on treatment decisions for patients in the persistent vegetative state. *Annual Report*, Appendix 7. BMA, London.

37. Emanuel, L.L., *et al.* (1991). Advance directives for medical care—case for greater use. *New England Journal of Medicine*, **324**, 889–95.

38. Gillick, M.R., Hesse, K., and Mazzapica, N. (1993). Medical technology at the end of life: what would physicians and nurses want for themselves? *Archives of Internal Medicine*, **153**, 2542–7.

39. Dyer, C. (1993). Law Lords rule that Tony Bland does not create a precedent. *British Medical Journal*, **306**, 413–14.

40. Tresch, D.D., *et al.* (1991). Patients in a persistent vegetative state: attitudes and reactions of family members. *Journal of the American Geriatrics Society*, **39**, 17–21.

41. Institute of Medical Ethics Working Party (1991). Report on withdrawing life supporting treatment from patients in a persistent vegetative state after acute brain damage. *Lancet*, **337**, 96–8.

42. Medical Council of New Zealand (1993). *Report from Bioethics Research Centre, University of Otago on persistent vegetative state and the withdrawal of food and fluids*. Medical Council of New Zealand, Wellington.

43. Gillon, R. (1993). Persistent vegetative state and withdrawal of nutrition and hydration. *Journal of Medical Ethics*, **19**, 67–8.

44. Gillon, R. (1993). Patients in the persistent vegetative state: a response to Dr Andrews. *British Medical Journal*, **306**, 1602–3.

45. Ahronheim, J.C. and Gasner, M.R. (1990). The sloganism of starvation. *Lancet*, **335**, 378–9.

46. Weir, R.F. and Gostin, L. (1990). Decisions to abate life-sustaining treatment for non-autonomous patients. *Journal of the American Medical Association*, **264**, 1846–53.

47. The Law Commission (1995). Mental incapacity (Report No. 231). HMSO, London.

48. The Scottish Law Commission (1995). Report on incapable adults (Report No. 151). Scottish Law Commission, Edinburgh.

49. House of Lords (1994). *Report of the Select Committee on Medical Ethics*. HL Paper 21.1. HMSO, London.

Consent to Treatment and Research in the ICU

J.K. Mason

It is probable that more ink has been spilled on the issue of consent than on any other aspect of medical jurisprudence. How, then, is one to say that consent to treatment and research in the intensive care unit (ICU) differs from that which has been the subject of so much discussion?

The answer that springs to mind immediately is that patients in the ICU are unconscious and are incapable of consent or dissent. This, however, is an over-simplification. It is true that a large proportion of patients in the unit will be there as a result of sudden and unexpected trauma—and, especially, head injury. But, at the other end of the scale, there are cases in which intensive care is an integral part of the therapeutic regime and where admission to the unit is, effectively, elective. The surprising feature of the ICU is, thus, not the uniformity but, rather, the diversity of the admissions. This is not to say that all units treat the same spread of patients. Depending on the size of the hospital complex, a number of specialist units may coexist. Whereas one unit may receive patients at the request of other departments—be they the accident and emergency department or the medical wards—the cardiovascular surgical department, for example, may follow its patients from admission for surgery, through treatment in its own intensive care unit to discharge. In short, one cannot even generalize the term 'ICU'; the clinical and ethical environments of each will differ one from another. It follows that all aspects of consent to treatment must be considered under what was, apparently, the specific heading of 'intensive care'.

1. The nature of consent

The law attaches great value to bodily privacy and physical integrity:

The existence of the patient's right to make his own decisions ... may be seen as a basic human right protected by the common law.[1]

Subject to a necessary application of the *de minimis* rule, which would include exempting 'physical contact which is generally accepted in the ordinary conduct of daily life',[2] any unwanted touching comes within the ambit of criminal battery or of the tort of trespass to the person, both of which are subsumed under the heading of assault in Scotland. Within the medical context, this has been well expressed in the oft-quoted words of the American Judge Cardozo, who said:

Every human being of adult years and sound mind has a right to determine what shall be done with his own body; and a surgeon who performs an operation without the patient's consent commits an assault[3]

Thus, it is the consent of the patient that legalizes the whole of medical examination and treatment and it is this which makes it such an important issue.

Treatment for which consent is given can be spoken of as voluntary therapy. Treatment of this type must be comparatively rare in the ICU and confined to those patients of whom it is known they will require intensive care, such as the elective cardiac surgical patient, or those who are subject to frequent admission due to, say, chronic respiratory disease. We will return to them in a brief discussion of informed consent (see p.38). At the other end of the scale, we have involuntary therapy that includes treatment for which there was no consent or which was positively rejected by the patient. With the possible exception of the attempted suicide—a matter referred to below—involuntary treatment of a competent adult can never be condoned and is always likely to attract litigation. As Lord Justice Butler-Sloss remarked in *Re T*: 'Doctors, therefore, who treat . . . a patient against his known wishes do so at their peril'.[4] This does not apply in the case of children represented by proxies, of whom it was said in a well-known American case:

People may be free to become martyrs themselves. But it does not follow that they are free in identical circumstances to make martyrs of their children.[5]

and, as for children themselves, an English judge has commented:

There is compelling and overwhelming force in the submission . . . that this court . . . should be very slow to allow an infant to martyr himself.[6]

Between these two extremes we have non-voluntary treatment—the need for which arises when the patient is, or is deemed to be, incapable of giving consent and when, as a result, his or her agreement to treatment must be assumed. The majority of such cases will derive from minors, the mentally incompetent, or the unconscious. It is this last type of case that will confront the intensive care practitioner most often and which is the main concern of this chapter. Even so, the problem of consent by children will also arise frequently and must be addressed as an issue in its own right.

Can consent be given?

The first question is, therefore, can consent be given?—and we must consider the inherent limitations to consent and how these can be accommodated within a legal and ethical framework of medical practice.

First, we must look at the legal restraints although these have very little relevance to the ICU. Obviously, there has to be a limitation on public policy grounds as to how much damage can be done to a person yet can be rendered blameless by reason of that person's consent to injury. This concern was well expressed over half a century ago:

As a general rule to which there are well established exceptions, it is an unlawful act to beat another person with such a degree of violence that the infliction of bodily harm is a probable consequence and, when such an act is proved, consent is immaterial.[7]

The fact that the surgeon's knife could be included within the exceptions to this rule was confirmed in *Attorney General's Reference (No 6 of 1980)*,[8] which referred specifically to reasonable surgical operations. It will be noted, however, that some control is still exercised. Some forms of 'cosmetic' surgery, such as non-therapeutic castration, might still be barred and the live donation of an organ that was essential to life would certainly be classified as unreasonable. Such considerations are, however, of academic interest only in the present context. We are here concerned primarily with the conditions that render non-voluntary treatment legally and ethically acceptable.

2. Non-voluntary treatment

The minor
The incompetent child. A child who is incapable of understanding the significance of a medical or surgical procedure is, by definition, incapable of consenting to its being applied to him or her. In these circumstances, the proxy consent of the parents or guardian renders medical or surgical intervention lawful. This is subject to what might be described as the 'reasonable parent' test. That is to say that the parents' consent—or withholding of consent—must be reasonable which, for this purpose, implies 'in the interests of the child'. Generally speaking, admission of a young child to intensive care involves no legal or ethical problems—the parents are competent to provide the necessary consent. Concern arises only when there is conflict between the parents and the medical advisers—or, put another way, only when the doctors regard the parents as acting unreasonably.

The procedure open to the health carers in such circumstances is now governed in England and Wales by the Children Act 1989. The Act restricts the use of wardship as a way of protecting a child against unreasonable parents and makes it clear that, in the majority of cases, the correct procedure for health carers who consider a child to be at risk is to apply for a care order under section 31 of the Act; the comparable authority in Scotland would be the Social Work (Scotland) Act 1968, section 44. In either case, a successful application would allow the local authority to assume responsibility for proxy decision-making on behalf of the child. In an emergency, however, this process might be too cumbersome and an alternative would be to invite the court to make a specific issue order under section 8(1) or to exercise its inherent jurisdiction on behalf of the Crown, which is very wide in the context of children.[9] Which of these is to be preferred is currently unclear;[10] it depends on the subtle interpretation of the limitations of statute and is of no concern to the doctor—in either case, the result will be in the form of an order or declaration by the court as to the procedure to be adopted. The courts have, recently, shown themselves remarkably sympathetic to the exercise of clinical judgement—including giving support to decisions not to institute intensive care, when not to do so was thought to be in the best interests of the sick child.[11] The interests of the child are paramount[12] and it may be in his or her best interests to be allowed to end life peacefully; the courts will not, however, countenance any suggestion of euthanasia—or the deliberate ending of life.

The mature minor.　It has been widely appreciated since the celebrated case of *Gillick*[13] that a minor does not become adult on a given date, rather:

parental right yields to the child's right to make his own decisions when he reaches a sufficient understanding and intelligence to be capable of making up his own mind on the matter requiring decision.[14]

and this applies, particularly, to medical treatment. The conditions enabling the doctor to decide whether or not a child below the age of 16 has attained the necessary intellectual maturity—as extrapolated from the specific problem of consent to contraceptive advice—were addressed by Lord Fraser in *Gillick*. Following this, Lord Donaldson coined the phrase '*Gillick*-competent' to describe the minor below the age of 16 years whose consent to medical treatment would be legally valid.[15] It is clear that the doctor may have considerable difficulty in deciding the presence or absence of '*Gillick*-competence' but it is a problem that is unlikely to arise in the context of intensive care. The parents will be able to consent on behalf of an unconscious minor, mature or not, as discussed in greater detail below.

The 16 to 18-year-old.　Consent by the minor aged 16 to 18 is covered in England and Wales by the Family Law Reform Act 1969, s.8(1) which states:

The consent of a minor who has attained the age of sixteen years to any surgical, medical or dental treatment which, in the absence of consent, would constitute a trespass to his person, shall be as effective as it would be if he were of full age; and where a minor has by virtue of this section given an effective consent to any treatment it shall not be necessary to obtain any consent for it from his parent or guardian . . .

Thus, from the point of view of the unconscious patient, or from that of the conscious patient likely to require elective intensive therapy, the minor over the age of 16 may be managed as if he or she was adult (see below)—and this applies throughout the UK.[16] Nevertheless, it is comforting to have effective consent if it can be obtained and there is now good authority that this can be given by the parents for any minor below the age of 18.

The basis for this lies in the twin 'consent' cases of *Re R*[17] and *Re W*[18] which caused a storm of academic protest when they were decided; the former concerned a '*Gillick*-competent' minor and the latter a girl aged 16. Both resulted in the court overruling an apparent rejection of treatment by the minor and, as such, were admittedly controversial. The decisions are, however, very helpful in the context of the intensive care unit as they provide an alternative route to legal consent to treatment. In *Re R*, the Master of the Rolls interpreted the decision in *Gillick* as eliminating only the right of the parents to *determine* the treatment of a mature child. He considered that the parental right to *consent* remained intact. This did not mean that treatment would necessarily be carried out—the wishes of a dissenting minor were to be given great weight—but it enabled the doctors to act if they thought it essential. *Re W* involved the interpretation of statute. The Family Law Reform Act 1969, s.8(3) qualifies s.8(1) in saying:

Nothing in this section [8(1)] shall be construed as making ineffective any consent which would have been effective if this section had not been enacted.

The majority of commentators have interpreted this as doing no more than consolidate the pre-existing common law right of the intelligent minor to consent on his or her own behalf.[19] The Master of the Rolls, however, saw it as preserving the parental right to consent which must have existed before the Act was passed.[20] If this interpretation is correct, there can be no doubt as to the parental position although the caveat as to the importance of a parallel refusal by the minor would apply with even greater force than in the case of the younger child. In maintaining a double source of legally acceptable consent to treatment of the mature minor, Lord Donaldson was clearly concerned with the interests of the medical profession—he spoke of consent as a protective 'flak-jacket' against litigation. This does very little for the recognition of children's rights to self-determination but it is of positive legal assistance to those involved in their treatment when they are unconscious, which is our main concern in the present context.

In passing, it may be observed that the inherent jurisdiction of the court can override statute—be it the Family Law Reform Act or the Children Act—in the case of persons aged less than 18 and this is irrespective of the minor's ability to make a reasoned decision. The court's powers extend beyond those of the natural parents and are, theoretically, limitless.[21] This *may* be so in Scotland but it is very unlikely that they would be invoked in similar circumstances.[22]

The mentally incapacitated

The most important new factor introduced under this heading is that, starting with the Mental Health Act 1959, current English mental health legislation has swept away the *parens patriae* jurisdiction—or the power of the state through its courts to intervene on behalf of its vulnerable citizens; the result is that no one now has the authority to *consent* to treatment on behalf of a mentally incompetent adult.[23] The Mental Health Act 1983[24] authorizes non-consensual treatment for the involuntary mental patient but only such treatment as relates directly to the mental condition; the Enduring Powers of Attorney Act 1985 makes no provision for the medical control of an incompetent and nor does the equivalent Law Reform (Miscellaneous Provisions) (Scotland) Act 1990, s.71. The result is a serious lacuna in the treatment of the mentally incapacitated which has given rise to judicial appeals for the restoration of the prerogative powers;[25] the Law Commission is currently studying the problem.[26]

This is not, however, to say that the court is powerless. The accepted practice when confronted with a treatment decision involving an incompetent patient—whether this be by virtue of mental incapacity or of unconsciousness due to disease or injury—is for the court to declare that a given treatment schedule will not be unlawful;[27] this exonerates the health care team from any future civil litigation.[28] In addition, the courts have, in many ways, delegated their powers to the medical profession. Thus, a declaration will not be needed when an apparently controversial result (e.g. sterilization), results from an action taken on acceptable clinical grounds (e.g. hysterectomy for intractable menorrhagia);[29] indeed, on occasion, the court has refused to make a declaration, not because it disagreed with the proposed course of treatment but because to do so might make other doctors think it was essential to obtain a court ruling in the circumstances.[30] Finally, the House of Lords has pointed to the practicalities of the situation—the whole process of providing health care for the mentally disabled would grind to a halt if a declaration from the courts was needed every time a surgical or dental operation was indicated for a mentally incompetent person.[31] This, then, brings us to a consideration of the common law as exemplified by the legal principle of necessity.

The unconscious adult

Just as no one can give consent on behalf of the mental patient, so no one, not even the court, can give consent on behalf of the unconscious, albeit previously competent, adult. The doctor who treats in such circumstances and in the absence of a declaration by the court relies on the common law principle of necessity. In simple terms, this means that acting unlawfully is justified if the resultant good effect materially outweighs the consequences of adhering strictly to the law. In Scotland, one could add in the civil law provision of *negotiorum gestio* which, again simplistically, means that a person who is incapacitated would expect others to do their best for him. The courts will take an extremely sympathetic view of the doctor who, despite having no formal consent, acts in the best interests of his patient—indeed, it has been indicated that he may have a common law duty to do so.[32] Moreover, whether or not the best interests were being served would be measured in *Bolam*[33] terms (see p. 39) which is, essentially, a judgment based on acceptable medical practice. The 'best interests' criterion is, however, crucial. In the present writer's opinion, there must be some doubt as to whether the court would consider it satisfied if non-consensual intensive care were given, say, to a dying patient for the sole purpose of providing donor organs for transplantation—and it is still more doubtful if close relatives could lawfully give permission for such a procedure while the patient was still alive[34] (see Chapter 10 for further discussion).

As an alternative to recourse to necessity—or to some form of *negotiorum gestio*—the doctor treating an unconscious patient might assume that he or she would consent if able to do so. Although this may, generally, be an arguable proposition, it is not a panacea. In some circumstances, the ICU will be faced with patients in whom such an assumption is by no means self-evident. Foremost among these are the uncompleted suicides which provide a substantial proportion of a unit's admissions. There is no certainty that all such cases represent parasuicides or *cris de coeur* and the health carer's dilemma is not eased by one of the more difficult passages from Lord Donaldson when Master of the Rolls. In discussing the possibility of a change of attitude to a previous rejection of medical treatment by an unconscious patient—which would include the would-be suicide—he had this to say:

> ... what the doctors *cannot* do is to conclude that, if the patient still had the necessary capacity in the changed situation [he being now unable to communicate], he would have reversed his decision ... What they *can* do is to consider whether at the time the decision was made it was intended by the patient to apply in the changed situation.[35]

Certainly, the majority of those responsible for the management of drug overdosage would act, unwittingly, on the basis of the former assumption; the latter seems to involve a degree of second guessing which is scarcely acceptable. Thus, the possibility of an action for battery or for trespass to the person on the part of a salvaged subject of attempted suicide is not as remote as might be thought—and it could be very real in the event that recovery resulted in a diminished quality of life.

However, although the possibility of an action exists, the chances of its success are, it is felt, minimal. There is no doubt that some element of evil intent would be essential before a charge of criminal assault would be accepted in Scotland and, in the civil law context, to attempt to attribute *culpa* to a medical team striving to save the life of a depressive patient borders on the bizarre. The situation in England is less certain. There is some suggestion that a non-consensual touching can be viewed as a battery in the absence of any hostile intent. The case commonly quoted as substantiating this premise is, however, unconvincing as a general authority;[36] the requirement for hostility voiced in *Wilson* v. *Pringle*[37] is more persuasive—and, incidentally, of more recent origin. It is almost certain that the court would be influenced by the antithesis of hostility evidenced by well-intentioned medical intervention and that no criminal liability would be attached. An action in tort for trespass would be equally available and it must not be forgotten that 'the Good Samaritan is a character unesteemed in English law'.[38] Moreover, the concept of the state's interest in preventing suicide, which is well-developed in the US,[39] has no comparable authoritative backing in the UK. Even so, despite the current antipathy to deciding cases on policy grounds, it is most unlikely that the courts would award damages against a doctor who intervened in a suicide attempt for just such reasons.[40] Skegg[41] specifically isolated some cases of attempted suicide from those cases in which refusal of consent releases a doctor from any obligation he or she would be under to save a patient's life. His reasons for doing so are not entirely clear and depend to an extent on a hopeful assumption that the patient would be glad of the intervention. Nevertheless, one can surely agree with him that, were the conduct of the intervening doctors to be questioned, the courts would hold it to be justified.

An associated, and perhaps more common, limitation on the plea of necessity rests on the immediacy of the need. It is a well-established principle that action in the absence of consent is justified only if it cannot be delayed until the patient is in a position to provide the necessary authority. This is illustrated in two well-known Canadian cases. In the first of these[42], a surgeon removed a testis during an operation for repair of a hernia; he pleaded successfully that the action was essential to the success of the operation and that, had he not acted so, the patient's health and life would have been imperilled because the testis was, itself, diseased. In the second[43], the surgeon performing a Caesarean section considered that the state of the uterus was such that a further pregnancy was medically undesirable; he, accordingly, tied the Fallopian tubes. He was successfully sued, the court taking the view that sterilization could and should have been postponed until the patient was in a position to make her own choice. Such situations are unlikely to occur in the ambience of intensive care; nevertheless, the general rule should be that the only 'necessary' treatment is that designed to return the patient to the state he or she was in before the emergency.

The value of an advance directive, popularly known as a 'living will', as an indication of the patient's attitude to intensive care when competent is very considerable in the US where the legal force of such documents is supported by statute in many states. Their special significance derives from the widespread application in the US of a 'substituted judgment' test—as opposed to a 'best interests' test—of the lawfulness of non-voluntary treatment. In the former test, the clinician attempts to assess what would have been the *patient's* likely response to the offer of intensive care and, clearly, the existence of a written directive greatly eases the task. The matter is discussed in detail in Chapter 5. Here it need only be said for the sake of completeness that advanced directives have, at present, no legal force in the UK but might, as in the case of relatives' agreement, strengthen the arm of the clinician faced with a difficult treatment decision. There is, in fact, evidence that at least some members of the House of

Lords are preparing to shift towards the American position; both Lord Keith and, more reservedly, Lord Goff in *Bland* appeared to see the advance directive as a legally valid expression of consent to or refusal of intensive care.[44]

In summary, treatment of the unconscious but previously competent adult is governed by a paradox. On the one hand, treatment without consent will constitute a civil wrong and might well be a crime. On the other, contrary to popular belief, no one, and certainly not the next-of-kin, has a legal right to consent or refuse treatment on behalf of the patient[45]. Consultation with relatives is almost always good medical practice and discussion may assist the clinician in coming to a therapeutic decision. At the end of the day, however, the physician's right to intervene depends on the common law; the patient's best interests provide the overriding measure of the legitimate extent of that intervention.

3. The conscious and competent adult

We are left, then, with the competent adult who must, as already discussed, be a relatively rare patient in the intensive care unit. None the less, they do occur; moreover, parents making decisions on behalf of their children do so as adults and must be treated as such. A short appraisal of the form of valid consent is, therefore, not out of place.

How is consent given?

Leaving aside the question of implied consent—which can have no place in such a serious matter as intensive care—valid consent may be given orally or in writing. Although both have the same jurisprudential value, the latter obviously gives greater protection to the doctor in the event of later conflict and should always be obtained when invasive surgery or anaesthesia is contemplated. Even so, the precise form of written consent is important and is becoming increasingly so. Thus, an American judge said of the common type of printed consent form (which is often couched in such terms as, 'I hereby give permission for myself to have a general anaesthetic and any operation the surgeon considers necessary'):

The so-called authority is so ambiguous as to be almost completely worthless.[46]

An echo of this sentiment was seen in the English case of *Chatterton* v. *Gerson*[47] where the implication was that, at most, such 'consent' would protect a surgeon in an action for battery. This, it is suggested, would apply even though it was agreed that 'the nature and purpose of the operation' had been explained. A more detailed form has now been produced for use in the National Health Service[48] which, at least to this writer, seems to express a co-operative doctor–patient relationship far better.

There is evidence to suggest that up to 44 per cent of post-operative patients who had completed the old type of form were unaware of the exact nature of the procedure they had undergone[49]. It is figures such as these that have catalysed the concept of informed consent.

Informed consent

The concept of informed consent derives from an increasing appreciation of the patient's autonomy, or right to self-determination. Applying this principle, the patient is no longer confined to acceptance or refusal of treatment that is offered; he or she should be allowed to choose the type and scope of treatment and to base this choice on adequate information as to success rates, risks, and the like. As it was put in US court:

A physician owes to his patient the duty to disclose in a reasonable manner all significant information that the physician possesses or reasonably should possess that is material to an intelligent decision by the patient whether to undergo the proposed procedure.[50]

It will be seen that failure to provide information may result in a breach of duty of care. Failure to inform thus falls within the tort of negligence for which the doctor may be liable if harm results. The injured patient is effectively saying: 'But for your failure to inform me of the risk, I would not have had the operation. As it was, I underwent the operation and the risk materialized. I have sustained damage and the fault is yours'.

Therefore, the basis for causation (i.e. the relationship between the doctor's action and the damage sustained) is clear. The difficulty lies in the interpretation of 'reasonable' and similar words and this, in turn, depends on whether they are viewed from the perspective of the patient or the doctor; accordingly, when considering the extent and the quality of the information that should be provided, we can think in terms of a standard based on the patient's expectations or of a professional standard.

A patient standard can be related to the subjective individual or to the objective, 'prudent' patient. The subjective patient test seeks to define what the *actual* plaintiff would have expected. It suffers from being very easily influenced by hindsight and, since the facts exist only in the mind of the individual, an accusation is very hard to refute. It is, however, a desirable standard in so far as it embodies personal factors, including many that are non-medical, which might affect a *particular* person's decision. Against this, under the prudent patient test, a plaintiff must establish that a *reasonable* person would not have chosen to undergo a recommended procedure after being advised of all significant risks. Although this suffers from the near impossibility of defining a 'reasonable patient' within the specific boundaries of each case, it is, in general, fair to both sides in that a reasonable doctor and a reasonable patient are meeting on comparable terms. It is the standard which is gradually taking over in the US.[51] The physician will, however, almost always be granted 'therapeutic privilege', that is to say, he may withhold information which, if imparted, would be detrimental to the health of the patient; this was also admitted by Lord Scarman in what was, effectively, a plea in the House of Lords for the acceptance of a patient standard in the UK.[52]

The professional standard, in contrast, measures what the reasonable doctor would be expected to tell the patient. It has been suggested that to follow a professional standard is advantageous as it leads to uniformity of judicial decisions and its adoption sounds unexceptional. That is, until it is appreciated that it is measured by the *Bolam* principle which is that: 'a doctor is not guilty of negligence if he has acted in accordance with a practice accepted as proper by a responsible body of medical men skilled in that particular art'.[53] The patient is, therefore, in difficulties. He or she can produce evidence that a majority of practitioners would not have done as the defendant did but this is to no avail if it can be shown that a responsible minority thought otherwise—and the judge cannot choose his preferred option.[54] Attempts have been made to soften the effects of *Bolam*[55] but none have been successful in the UK[56] where the doctrine shows every sign of survival.[57] In contrast, the *Bolam* principle, as regards consent is under attack in other common law jurisdictions—it is fast disappearing in the US, it has been rejected in Canada, and it has received a death blow in Australia.[58]

The plaintiff in consent-based negligence cases faces other, more indefinite, problems. In particular, the two parties are unlikely to be evenly balanced in their abilities to remember discussions and their contained semantic niceties. There is small wonder that successful actions are so rare, so much so that I have only found reports of two such cases, neither of which sets an entirely satisfactory precedent.[59]

The concept of informed consent is firmly fixed in medical minds and is referred to frequently in the medical press. It is, therefore, interesting to find such authoritative legal comments as:

The doctrine of informed consent has no place in English law.[60]

or

English law does not accept the transatlantic concept of informed consent.[61]

or, in Scotland:

as I see it, the law in both Scotland and England has come down firmly against the view that the doctor's duty to the patient involves at all costs obtaining the informed consent of the patient to specific medical treatments.[62]

Clearly, there is scope for misunderstanding. The judges were, in fact, referring to informed consent as judged by either the subjective or reasonable patient standard. The patient's need for sufficient information on which to make a truly valid consent still applies in the UK. The true state of the current law was probably best summed up by Lord Templeman:

The patient is free to decide whether or not to submit to treatment recommended by the doctor and therefore the doctor impliedly contracts to provide information which is adequate to enable the patient to reach a balanced judgment.[63]

4. Refusal of treatment

Given the importance of consent in the practice of medicine, is there a corresponding positive right to refuse treatment as opposed to a negative right to withhold consent? The UK has, perhaps, lagged behind other common law jurisdictions in this respect. A common law right of 'informed refusal' is now well established in the US and this clearly applies to patients in intensive care.[64] Refusal of treatment is recognized in the Canadian Charter of Rights and Freedom.[65] and, in Australia, Victoria has the Medical Treatment Act 1988, which not only gives a statutory right to the patient to refuse treatment but also introduces the offence of medical trespass that is committed by a practitioner who gives treatment contrary to the certified wishes of the patient; at the same time, the Act exonerates the doctor who omits to treat on these grounds from civil or criminal liability. There is, however, no doubt that a common law right of refusal exists both in England and Wales and in Scotland and this has been confirmed in two relatively recent cases.[66] Great importance is placed, rightly, on the mental capacity to refuse and on the absence of coercion when doing so. The tenor of the decision in *Re T*, which involved an adult Jehovah's Witness who was strongly influenced by her mother, indicates that the patient may have to prove this to the satisfaction of the doctor concerned. This judgment, however, rested on the facts of the particular case; as a general rule, the warning note sounded by Lord Justice Staughton,

I cannot find authority that the decision of a doctor as to the existence or refusal of consent is sufficient protection [against civil action] if the law subsequently decides otherwise[67]

should be heeded. It clearly indicates that the court should be consulted in any difficult case.

Since the validity of refusal is grounded in capacity, minors must be considered as a separate concern. The child who is too young to understand may refuse treatment through its parents or guardian; this, however, would be subject to the 'reasonable parent' test discussed above. Thus, refusal of a blood transfusion on behalf of an infant might well not—indeed, almost certainly would not—be regarded as reasonable; on the other hand, decisions as to the treatment, and especially as to intensive treatment, of severe physical deformity in the newborn can be, and very frequently are, taken by parents in consultation with the doctors involved.[68] Whether the right to consent to treatment vested in the *Gillick*-competent minor and the minor aged 16–18 years carries with it a right to refuse treatment has been a matter for debate since *Re R* and *Re W*[69] were decided. The majority of commentators believe that it does—it even being suggested that it borders on the perverse to hold otherwise.[70] The present writer agrees that the *capacity* exists but that, in the case of *Gillick*-competence, the measurement of that capacity differs. Thus, it is one thing to have the understanding to accept the advice of a trained professional; it is quite another for a 15-year-old, effectively, to claim superior medical intelligence to that of an experienced physician or surgeon.[71] The *right* to do so may be present equally but the *degree* of understanding needed to satisfy Lord Fraser's test in *Gillick*[72] must be different. The current concepts of parallel parental rights to consent apply to both types of mature minor as discussed above; there are, however, no comparable parental rights of refusal in the face of consent by the minor.

5. Consent and withdrawal of treatment

Withdrawal of intensive care can be justified on more than one count. On clinical grounds, it is clear that a productive–non-productive treatment test can be applied (i.e. that treatment of any sort, including life-sustaining treatment, can be withdrawn when it is producing no useful result).[73] The decision must, however, be based on concern for the individual patient alone. Lord Justice Balcombe, in emphasizing that the court should not dictate a form of treatment to reluctant doctors, said:

the effect of [an order such as was given] might have been to require the health authority to put [the child] on a ventilator in an intensive care unit, and thereby possibly to deny the benefit of those limited resources to a child who was much more likely . . . to benefit from them.[74]

I interpret this as meaning that, while the law accepts that a choice may be made between two persons seeking *admission* to intensive care, it would not approve *removal* of a patient simply because of the arrival of a more deserving case; the only permissible bench-mark would be the status of the patient already under treatment. It would then be possible to look at withdrawal within a consent context. The common thread of the Law Lords' opinions in *Bland*[75] was that a patient—who, in the case of a minor, would be the patient's proxy—had a right to refuse treatment and that he or she should not be deprived of that right by reason of incompetence. There were clearly times when the patient, if able, would say: 'I have had enough. I retract my consent'. The House was, therefore, effectively prepared to apply a 'substituted judgment' test, albeit being determined to dress this up in the language of the welfare principle,[76] and this would provide a general line of justification on both ethical and clinical grounds.

Even so, the agreement of the relatives may be difficult to obtain, especially when withdrawal of treatment is expressed in terms implying 'switching off the machine'. In point of fact, patients who have reached the non-productive phase of intensive care are generally surviving only by virtue of the drugs and other therapies that are ancillary to mechanical ventilation; withdrawal of the former results in a quiet and painless death which avoids a highly emotional action and is far more acceptable to the grieving relatives.

Finally, the intensivist cannot ignore the economics of his calling. It costs approximately £1250 per day to maintain a patient in a high-grade intensive care unit. By consenting to treatment, even if only by way of necessity, the patient does not acquire a right to treatment of every form; and, on the other side of the coin, it is clearly wrong to drain the National Health Service of such resources on behalf of a patient who cannot benefit from them.[77]

6. Research in the ICU

It is generally agreed that conditions validating consent to research or experimentation must be that much more strict than they are in the case of therapy (e.g. no relaxations such as 'therapeutic privilege' are permissible). For the purposes of this section, we can assume that no potential research subjects in the ICU will be capable of consent; it follows that justification of research can only be by way of necessity and this may be very hard to establish. Indeed, in this writer's opinion, research on unconscious patients which was not directed to the well-being of unconscious patients, either as a group or as individuals, could not be undertaken unless it was both anonymous and non-invasive.

On the other hand, intensive treatment is unlikely to be improved without research on actual patients and it could, as a result, be seen to lie within the mantle of necessity—but the degree of protection provided would be limited. Save in exceptional circumstances, it would, for example, be unethical to insert another intravascular line purely for research purposes; invasive procedures that would not normally be carried out would be very difficult to justify. Therapeutic research in a non-voluntary group would need to have been particularly well evaluated in animals or consenting humans, and the need for randomization would also need special consideration. Perhaps of greatest importance is that any research project involving bodily invasion, risk, or alteration of an established and accepted regime would have to be approved by a research ethics committee.[78] The agreement of close relatives might be appropriate in some cases but, as we have seen, it has no legal effect when the subjects are adults. In such circumstances, to place extra stress on those who may already be distraught could be seen as being not merely unnecessary but actually contraindicated.[79]

A distinction can be made between research, which implies regulation by a strict, prefabricated protocol, and a purposeful search for knowledge, and experimental or innovative treatment which is, generally, unplanned and directed to the interests of the individual patient. The two categories often overlap—an innovative treatment might, for example, be used for a small group of similar patients—but their separation is useful in so far as previously unexplored treatment may well be indicated in what *The Lancet* has called an 'ethical emergency'.[80] In a probable scenario, there will be insufficient time to convene and consult an ethics committee and the physician will be acting on his own initiative. Authority for his so doing is to be found in the Declaration of Helsinki,[81] which approves the free use of new diagnostic measures that offer 'hope of saving life, re-establishing health, or alleviating suffering'—the characteristic remit of the intensive care unit. At the end of the day, however, the morality of any medical procedure depends not so much on academic declarations—nor, indeed, on the letter of the law—but, rather, on how the doctor's actions will appear in the eyes of his peers. In this respect, it should not be forgotten that intensive care is intensive not only for the patient but also for the health carers involved.

Acknowledgement

I am grateful to Dr A. Pollock, Royal Infirmary, Edinburgh for a most helpful briefing on the organization of an intensive care unit.

Notes

1. *Sidaway* v. *Bethlem Royal Hospital Governors* (1985). 1 BMLR 132 per Lord Scarman, p. 140.
2. *Collins* v. *Wilcock* (1984). 79 Cr App R 229 per Goff LJ, p. 234.
3. *Schloendorff* v. *Society of New York Hospital* 105 NE 92 (NY, 1914), p. 93.
4. *Re T (adult: refusal of treatment)* (1992) 9 BMLR 46 p. 63.
5. *Prince* v. *Massachusetts* 321 US Rep 158 (1944).
6. *Re E (a minor)* (1992) 9 BMLR 1 per Ward J, p. 9.
7. *R* v. *Donovan* [1934] 2 KB 498 per Swift J, p. 507. The principle has been endorsed in *R* v. *Brown and others* [1993] 2 All ER 75.
8. [1981] QB 715.
9. The route to the courts in Scotland would be by way of the Law Reform (Parent and Child) (Scotland) Act1986, s.3.
10. In *Re O (a minor) (medical treatment)* [1993] 2 FLR 149 the inherent jurisdiction of the High Court was preferred. In a later case *Re R (a minor) (blood transfusion)* [1993] 2 FCR 544, the judge opted for a specific issue order—stating that the inherent jurisdiction was always available as a back-up.
11. See *Re C (a minor) (wardship: medical treatment)* [1989] 2 All ER 782 (a terminally ill child); *Re J (a minor) (wardship: medical treatment)* (1990) 6 BMLR 25 (seriously, but not terminally, ill child).
12. Guardianship of Minors Act 1971, s.1.
13. *Gillick* v. *West Norfolk and Wisbech Area Health Authority* (1985) 2 BMLR 11, HL.
14. Per Lord Scarman at BMLR 35. Note that the principle of the mature minor is incorporated in Scots law into statute so far as medical treatment is concerned: Age of Legal Capacity (Scotland) Act 1991, ss.1(1)(b) and 2(4).
15. In *Re R (a minor) (wardship: medical treatment)* (1991) 7 BMLR 147, p. 155.
16. The Age of Legal Capacity (Scotland) Act 1991, s.1(1)(b) states very clearly that

a person of or over the age of 16 years shall have legal capacity to enter into any transaction. For discussion of the English and Scottish positions, see Edwards L. (1993). The right to consent and the right to refuse: More problems with minors and medical consent. *Juridical Review*, 52.

17. See note 15.

18. *Re W (a minor) (medical treatment)* (1992) 9 BMLR 22.

19. For example, see Gostin, L. (1992). Consent to treatment: The incapable person. In *Doctors, patients and the law*, (ed. C. Dgen), p. 75. Blackwell Scientific Publications, Oxford.

20. The present writer has always supported this view—but it is certainly not that accepted by the House of Lords in *Gillick*. There were persistent efforts to categorize Lord Donaldson's views on parental rights as *obiter*—or not binding—but he chose *Re W* as a vehicle by which to re-emphasize the significance of his remarks in *Re R*.

21. *Re W*, see note 18, per Lord Donaldson, p. 33. Confirmed in *South Glamorgan County Council* v. *B and W* (1992) 11 BMLR 162, p. 171.

22. For a discussion, see Edwards, note 16.

23. *F* v. *West Berkshire Health Authoirty* (1989) 4 BMLR 1 per Lord Brandon, p. 10.

24. And its counterpart, the Mental Health (Scotland) Act 1984.

25. For example, *F (Mental patient) (Sterilisation)* (1988) 138 NLJ LR 150 per Scott Baker J, p. 151; *T* v. *T* [1988] Fam 52 per Wood, J., p. 68.

26. Law Commission (1993). Mentally incapacitated adults and decision-making. Consultation paper no. 129. For resumé, see Brahams, D. (1993). Consent to research in presence of incapacity. *Lancet*, **341**, 1143.

27. Controlled by Rules of the Supreme Court, Order 15, Rule 16.

28. Although it can have little, if any, relevance in the context of intensive care, this may not be so in respect of criminal proceedings: *Imperial Tobacco Ltd* v. *Attorney-General* [1980] 1 All ER 866.

29. See *F* v. *F* (1991) 7 BMLR 135.

30. *Re H (mental patient)* [1993] 4 Med LR 91.

31. *F* v. *West Berkshire Health Authority*, note 23, per Lord Brandon, p. 8.

32. Note 31, per Lord Brandon.

33. *Bolam* v. *Friern Hospital Management Committee* (1957) 1 BMLR 1 per Lords Brandon, Giffiths, and Goff in *F*, note 23, pp. 19, 20, 27.

34. Authority to consent to donation materializes under the Human Tissue Act 1961 only after death.

35. *Re T*, note 4, p. 60.

36. *Collins* v. *Wilcock*, note 2.

37. [1986] 2 All ER 440.

38. Lord Devlin, P. (1962). *Samples of law making*, p. 90. Oxford University Press. The topic was completely different but the words have a disturbing ring in the context of intensive care.

39. For example, see. *In re Guardianship of Grant* 747 P 2d 445 (Wash, 1987); *In the matter of Kathleen Farrell* 529 A 2d 404 (NJ, 1987).

40. See Butler-Sloss, L.J. (1988) in *Re T*, note 4.

41. Skegg, P.D.G. (1988) *Law, ethics, and medicine*, (rev. edn), pp. 110–16, 155–7. Clarendon Press, Oxford.

42. *Marshall* v. *Curry* [1993] 3 DLR 260.

43. *Murray* v. *McMurchy* [1949] 2 DLR 442.

44. *Airedale NHS Trust* v. *Bland* (1993) 12 BMLR 64 pp. 105, 112. Further confirmation of this view is to be found in *Re C (adult: refusal of treatment)* [1994] 1 All ER 819 per Thorpe, J., p. 824.

45. Per Lord Donaldson in *Re T*, note 4, p. 50.

46. *Rogers* v. *Lumbermens Mutual Cas Co* 119 So 2d 649 (La, 1960).

47. [1981] 1 All ER 257.

48. NHS Management Executive (1990). *A guide to consent for examination and treatment.*

49. Byrne, D.J., Napier, A., and Cuschieri, A. (1988). How informed is signed consent? *British Medical Journal*, **296**, 839

50. *Harnish* v. *Children's Hospital Medical Center* 439 NE 2d 240 (Mass, 1982). Note the use of the word 'intelligent'. The writer greatly prefers the use of some such word rather than 'informed'; information is useless unless it is understood.

51. For example, see *Largey* v. *Rothman* 540 A 2d 504 (NJ, 1988).

52. *Sidaway*, note 1, p. 145.

53. *Bolam*, note 33, per McNair J, p. 5.

54. *Maynard* v. *West Midlands Regional Health Authority* (1983) 1 BMLR 122.

55. In *Gold* v. *Haringey Health Authority* [1986] 1 FLR 125 the trial judge attempted to dissociate the principle from counselling; in *Hills* v. *Potter* [1984] 1 WLR 641, 'responsible' body was amended to 'both respectable and responsible' (p. 651); in *Sidaway* at the Appeal stage, the Master of the Rolls said the opinion should be '*rightly*' regarded as proper—the court being the arbiter: [1984] 1 All ER 1018.

56. The Scottish equivalent is *Hunter* v. *Hanley* 1955 SC 200. The cases are commonly cited together with approval.

57. Where its scope may even be widening. In *Blyth* v. *Bloomsbury Health Authority* [1993] 4 Med LR 151, Kerr LJ was prepared to consider extending the principle to answering specific enquiries.

58. *Reibl* v. *Hughes* (1980) DLR (3d) 1; *Rogers* v. *Whitaker* (1992) 109 ALR 625, [1993] 4 Med LR 79. For a comprehensive analysis of consent 'standards', see McLean, S.A.M. (1989) *A patient's right to know*. Dartmouth, Ardershot.

59. *Thake* v. *Maurice* (1986) 1 All ER 497; *Goorkani* v. *Tayside Health Board* 1991 SLT 94.

60. Per Dunn LJ in *Sidaway* [1984] 1 All ER 1018, CA, p. 1030.

61. Per Lord Donaldson MR in *Re T*, note 4, p. 61.

62. Per Lord Caplan in *Moyes* v. *Lothian Health Board* 1990 SLT 444, p. 449.

63. In *Sidaway*, note 1, p. 159.

64. *Bouvia* v. *The Superior Court of Los Angeles County* 179 Cal App 3d 1127 (1986); *Re Kathleen Farrell*, note 39; *Fossmire* v. *Nicoleau* 551 NE 2d 77 (NY, 1990).

65. S.7. But the right is not absolute and can be withdrawn in the public interest. See *Rodriguez* v. *Attorney General for Canada and Attorney General for British Columbia* (1993) 107 DLR (4d) 342.

66. *Re T* (1992), note 4. *Re C*, note 44, in which an injunction was given prohibiting a hospital amputating the leg of a schizophrenic who refused permission for the operation.

67. Note 4, p. 68.

68. For a particularly good outline of how such decisions are reached, see Laing, I.A. (1989). Withdrawing from invasive neonatal intensive care. In *Paediatric forensic medicine and pathology*, (ed. J.K. Mason), Ch. 8. Chapman & Hall, London.

69. Notes 16 and 19.

70. Kennedy, I. (1992). Consent to treatment: The capable person. In *Doctors, patients and the law*, (ed. C. Dyer). p. 61. Blackwell Scientific Publications, Oxford.

71. This seems to underly the decision in *Re C.* note 6, in which the court overruled the refusal of blood transfusion by a 15-year-old boy who was, admittedly, able to appreciate the consequences of his decision. Ward J said: 'I cannot discount at least the possibility that he may in later years suffer some diminution in his convictions' (p. 8).

72. Note 14, p. 24.

73. For discussion, see Mason, J.K. and McCall Smith, R.A. (1994). *Law and medical ethics*, (4th edn), p. 324. Butterworths, London.

74. *Re J (a minor) (wardship: medical treatment)* (1992) 9 BMLR 10 p. 20. The ventilator certainly cannot be occupied for a third party's convenience when the patient is dead: see *Re A* [1992] 3 Med LR 303.

75. *Airedale NHS Trust* v. *Bland* (1993) 12 BMLR 64. Now followed in *Frenchay Healthcare NHS Trust* v. *S.* [1994] 2 All ER 403.

76. I suggest that the reluctance of the English courts to apply a substituted judgment test stems from the test's close association with advance directives that have been develped in the US. The matter is discussed in Chapter 5.

77. It is to be noted that concern for the economics of intensive care was acknowledged in *Bland*, see note 75. See also Chapters 11 and 12.

78. See RCP (Royal College of Physicians) (1990). *Guidelines on the practice of ethics committees in medical research involving human subjects* (working party), (2nd edn). RCP, London.

79. See Tobias, J.S. and Souhami R.L. (1993). Fully informed consent can be needlessly cruel. *British Medical Journal*, **307**, 1199.

80. Editorial (1992). Ethical emergencies. *Lancet*, **339**, 399.

81. Para II.1. Reproduced as Appendix F in Mason and McCall Smith (1994), note 73.

4

Withholding and Withdrawing Medical Treatment

N. Pace

1. Introduction

The rapid progress made by medical technology is a two-edged sword.[1] Despite all the attendant benefits, its greater availability and use has presented medicine and society with unprecedented ethical, legal, and economic dilemmas. Nowhere is this more clearly demonstrated than in the intensive care unit (ICU). As a result of these advances, many patients who would have rapidly succumbed a few years ago can now be kept alive for much longer. In some cases, such as those patients who are in a persistent vegetative state (PVS), this can be many years. In particular, questions surrounding the withholding or withdrawing of treatment remain largely unanswered, especially in Britain.

In some situations, despite no apparent possibility of recovery, life may be sustained artificially and indefinitely by means of advanced techniques of life support because doctors, care givers, and patients (or their proxies) are not sure what their legal and ethical obligations are, a situation compounded by disagreement among doctors, ethicists, lawyers, and churchmen. For example, the Linacre Centre, a Roman Catholic institution, states:

When the patient's physical condition has become hopeless it is often appropriate, depending on the type of case, either to withdraw some of the treatment already instituted or, without stopping existing treatment, to cease instituting treatments for new disorders as they arise. Thus, depending on the case, it may be right, for example, to discontinue an infusion of cardiac stimulants, or to allow, say, renal failure, supervening on an already hopeless condition, to take its course without treating it . . . It may also be right to discontinue artificial pulmonary ventilation.[2]

Now consider the following extract from Campbell:[3]

Switching off a machine can be regarded as the abandonment of an attempt to restore life, since it has become clear that the process of dying cannot be reversed (although it might be arrested for an indefinite period). Removal of the support of the machine permits the process of dying to continue, if the patient is incapable of sustaining respiration spontaneously. For this reason, the action of switching off the machine can be regarded as permitting death rather than actively causing it. There is no way back to life as normally understood and no benefit to the patient in remaining indefinitely in a state of suspended dying. Critical to this argument is agreement that *cerebral death* is equivalent to the end of personal existence. This must be the *only reason* for switching it off.

Thus it would appear that there is some degree of disagreement between the two. Campbell would only allow withdrawal of treatment if the patient had suffered cerebral death. No mention is made of futile treatment or future quality of life. However, it is well known that treatment is regularly withheld or withdrawn from patients who are not cerebrally dead in hospitals throughout the world. Either Campbell is wrong in his assertion that treatment can only be withdrawn in cases of cerebral death, or doctors are behaving unethically and possibly illegally.

Doctors have a moral obligation to always act in the best interests of their patients, provided they keep within their own moral and ethical principles. However, they frequently attempt to prolong survival of patients in end-stage organ failure. Some of these patients have no prospect of returning to a reasonable quality of life. Death may be seen by them as a failure of their medical or surgical skills. If they merely prolong the inevitable and the patient is not allowed to die with dignity, then clearly, they are not acting in the patient's best interests. Often a fresh view may offer a better appreciation of where the patient's best interests lie.[4] The use of medical technology may therefore be inappropriate in several situations.

In a recent study from San Francisco, medical treatment was withheld from 22 and withdrawn from 93 patients out of a total of 1719 admissions into an ICU over a year.[5] The main reasons for not treating or stopping treatment were either brain death or poor prognosis. Other reasons mentioned were futility of further treatment, extreme suffering, and requests by the patient's family. Concern about resources was not given as a reason and neither was bed availability in the ICU.

It therefore appears that life support was withheld or withdrawn infrequently but clearly did occur. Mechanical ventilation was the treatment most frequently withdrawn and vasopressors the intervention most frequently withheld. 'Do not resuscitate' (DNR) orders preceded the actual withholding or withdrawing of further treatment and appeared to be a crucial point in the decision to limit treatment. The authors withheld or withdrew vasopressors as their first choice wherever possible, considering this to be the most humane way of withholding or withdrawing support.

Regarding mechanical ventilation, the authors stated:

As the initial step in withdrawing the ventilator, supplemental oxygen and positive end-expiratory pressure were usually discontinued. Patients were then placed on a T-piece only if these actions had not resulted in a quick death. There were no cases in which physicians or nurses insisted on continuing ventilation because it had been initiated; ... care givers believed that withdrawing treatment was as ethically appropriate as not starting it in the first place. Sedatives and analgesic drugs were frequently given to patients during this process to reduce air hunger.

It is well recognized that if mechanical ventilation is withheld, good medical practice requires any discomfort to be relieved, even at high doses which may hasten death.[6,7] However, decisions to withhold or withdraw treatment that may lead to the death of the patient appear to be against the principle to preserve life found in medical and legal tradition. Are doctors therefore compelled to offer a patient all available means at their disposal in order that his or her life is prolonged at all costs? Furthermore, are they allowed to administer drugs, such as morphine, to relieve discomfort despite the possibility of such drugs hastening death? An analysis of ethical and legal principles is required to answer these questions.

2. Ethical principles: sanctity of life

The 'sanctity of life' doctrine was universally accepted a few years ago. The rapid development of technology, however, appears to be gradually shifting the problem from the means to reversing the dying process to questions regarding the quality of life sustained and preserved.[8] Sometimes, the quality of the additional life gained can be so severely compromised that both the patient and his or her health carers may question the value of starting or continuing such therapy.

An extreme view of the sanctity of life doctrine would claim that survival is the sole objective of human existence and therefore clinical practice must be dominated by that objective. It manifests itself in such assertions as absolute priority must be given to life-threatening situations, and only when they have been dealt with should society worry about quality of life. This would mean taking resources away from activities which merely relieve pain and discomfort, or which merely increase people's functional capacity, and directing them instead into activities designed to stop people dying. Thus, most people living today would have to endure a great deal of unrelieved (but relievable) pain and suffering, with no one being permitted to die until everything that was possible had been tried (and had failed).[9]

This is unacceptable. Clearly, what is desired is not really life as such, but enjoyable and worthwhile experiences. Life itself has no intrinsic value. Life has value only if it is worth living. When there is no further scope for enjoyable or worthwhile experiences, mere continuing existence may not be worth having.

Rachels[10] points out that there is a major difference between 'having a life' and merely 'being alive'. Being alive is relatively unimportant. One's 'life', by contrast, is immensely important. It is the sum of one's aspirations, decisions, activities, projects, and human relationships. It is therefore persons, not all humans, whose lives have value. Unless there is a capacity for self-awareness, for the individual to recognize him or herself as a functioning human person able to relate to other persons, he or she has no life of the quality and kind which must be preserved.[11]

Medicine cannot have an unqualified interest in life. If this is to be the standard for medical decision-making, it distorts the very function of medicine, and misconstrues what makes medical decision-making good.[12] The whole point of medical practice is to improve (beneficence) or at least maintain (non-maleficence) a patient's quality of life. Thus, medicine cannot be practised with the goal being the unqualified interest in the preservation of life.

Some theologians have also accepted quality over sanctity. O'Donnell[13] notes that life is a relative, not an absolute good, and McCormick[8] states that life is not a value to be preserved in and for itself but:

It is a value to be preserved precisely as a condition for other values, and therefore in so far as these other values remain attainable.

Commenting on ICUs, Dunstan[14] claims that:

The success of intensive care is not ... to be measured only by the statistics of survival, as though each death were a medical failure. It is to be measured by the quality of the lives preserved or restored; and by the quality of the dying of those in whose interest it is to die; and by the quality of human relationships involved in each death.

The problem with quality of life is that it is difficult to define and quantify, and no definition is universally acceptable. 'Good' quality of life may mean different things to different people and, with the passage of time, the things that matter most may change. Health may be described in a variety of ways, but in an autonomous society this requires starting from ordinary people's own ideas about how they recognize ill-health, and what aspects of ill-health they are most anxious to avoid. This is considered in greater detail in Chapter 7.

It must be stressed, however, that quality of life judgements can never fully replace sanctity of life. Otherwise, visions of a 'slippery slope' arise. The senile, the elderly, the demented, the terminally ill, and handicapped newborns, who, it may be claimed, all have a lower quality of life than 'normal' human beings, will be condemned to death. They would appear to have a lower social worth and therefore less 'right to live'.

It is thus possible to recognize that human life deserves respect (i.e. accepting sanctity of life), whereas acknowledging that in some cases, such as the terminally ill or patients in a persistent vegetative state, a quality of life approach can supersede. The contention that prolonging life is always in the patient's interest is therefore rejected.[15] Furthermore, the Roman Catholic Church also affirms this position since it accepts (indeed instituted) the distinction between 'ordinary and extraordinary means'.[16]

3. Ordinary and extraordinary means

This distinction offers doctors and patients a reasonable and straightforward basis of assessing what is obligatory treatment, or what Gillon describes as 'how much to strive to keep alive'.[17]

Ordinary means have been defined as all medicines, treatments, and operations, which offer a reasonable hope of benefit for the patient and which can be obtained and used without excessive expense, pain, or other inconvenience. Extraordinary means are all medicines, treatments, and operations, which cannot be obtained or used without excessive expense, pain, or other inconvenience or which, if used, would not offer a reasonable hope of benefit.[18]

It is important to realize that, because of the rapid advances made by technology in the past few years, what is now ordinary may possibly not have been so a few years ago. Penicillin today is in common use in the treatment of a variety of infections and is highly likely to be considered 'ordinary' in the vast majority of cases.[3] Not so long ago it was not so readily available and probably constituted extraordinary treatment.

Others have claimed that it is better to refer to 'proportionate' and 'disproportionate' treatment or 'obligatory' and 'optional' treatment.[19] All the terms, however, are for practical purposes interchangeable. In summary, the distinction claims that the good of saving life is morally obligatory only if its pursuit is not excessively burdensome or disproportionate in relation to the expected benefits. Beauchamp and Childress[19] have further extended this argument by claiming that in certain situations, the burdens can so outweigh the benefits to the patient that the treatment is wrong rather than optional.

One of the major problems with the distinction is that the terms 'benefit' and 'burden' are open to interpretation.

The more difficult factors to assess in judging whether treatment is obligatory concern what is traditionally called the burdensome character of treatment. In judging how burdensome treatment is, consideration is to be given to the degree of risk, cost and physical and psychological hardship involved relative (a) to this particular patient, his overall condition and its potential for improvement, his resources and sensibilities, and (b) to this particular doctor (or medical team), his time, effort and other obligations.[2]

The criteria for assessing whether a proposed treatment is burdensome are, therefore, not precise and will differ depending on the circumstances of the patient. Similarly, individual doctors and, more importantly, individual patients will have different priorities. The situation is therefore similar to people's differences in evaluating quality of life.

Many will value the opportunity for human interaction above the mere absence of pain. This is highly relevant today because of ethical dilemmas regarding treatment of patients in a persistent vegetative state (PVS). Many would find being in this condition unacceptable, with loss of dignity and intellectual capability and being fully dependent on others for personal hygiene. The patient, however, cannot be said to be suffering because he or she is completely unaware. In this situation, the burdens appear to fall mainly on others, rather than the patient.[20]

It is accepted, therefore, that the distinction may not always resolve dilemmas and indeed, may lead to disagreement about the best course of action. What is clear is that decisions have to be based only on the information available at that particular time. Consider a particular disease which presently is invariably fatal. One cannot base one's decisions on the remote possibility that a cure may be found in ten years time. Medical therapy is either appropriate or inappropriate at any particular time and to try to predict the future is risky.[7]

If a distinction can feasibly be made between proportionate and disproportionate treatment, then any treatment may, in a particular situation, be deemed not to be morally obligatory. This must, therefore, also be the case for artificial feeding since the influential President's Commission,[21] the Hastings Centre[22] the American Medical Association,[23] and the British Medical Association all accept that artificially provided nutrition and hydration constitute medical treatment.

Ruark and Raffin[24] interestingly include supplemental oxygen among their basic life-support measures. Campbell[3] also believes that in terms of cost and availability, the administration of oxygen is certainly to be regarded as an ordinary means. This implies morally obligatory treatment. Supplemental oxygen has never featured highly in discussions about withdrawing treatment. From personal experience, doctors in ICUs are quite comfortable to withdraw supplemental oxygen and to ventilate a patient with air. Requesting them to stop giving fluids or even withdraw ventilation is a different matter altogether. It could be that doctors may be deluding themselves into believing that it is acceptable to withdraw oxygen but not ventilation because the patient does not die immediately when ventilated with air. The immediate causal link between death and stopping ventilation makes intensivists much more wary. It is perceived as directly killing the patient since the patient dies within a matter of minutes. This essentially is the crux of the 'acts and omissions' doctrine.

4. Acts and omissions

The 'acts and omissions' doctrine argues that actions that result in some undesirable consequence are, in general, morally worse than inactions, or failures to act, that have the same consequence. Such a doctrine appears appealing simply because people do not feel as morally responsible for their omissions as they do for their actions.

Thus, a positive action carries the presumption that the agent incurs responsibility for intentionally doing it. An omission, on the other hand, carries no such acceptance of responsibility.[2] In essence, the distinction argues that there is a difference between the act of killing and the omission of letting a patient die.

This distinction, however, can be criticized. Of prime importance is the observation that when one considers the intentions of the agent or the consequences of the action or omission, there seems to be no real difference at all.

In his often-quoted article on active and passive euthanasia, Rachels[25] shows that there can be no moral distinction between acts and omissions by offering the following example. Smith and Jones both stand to inherit fortunes if their six-year-old cousins die before them. Smith drowns one of his cousins in the bath, making it seem like an accident. Jones intends to drown his cousin in the bath but on creeping up on him in the bathroom sees the boy slip, bang his head, and slide unconscious beneath the water. Jones waits to make sure that the boy really does die and is ready to push his head back under the water if he should surface, but the boy drowns accidentally.

The two cases are identical apart from the fact that one is a case of an act and one is a case of an omission. Rachels therefore argues that no one would claim that there is any moral difference between the two cases. In particular, he claims Jones is as morally culpable as Smith, both acting from the same motive, and in both cases the consequences are identical. He concludes, therefore, that in the absence of other morally important differences the bare distinction between acts and omissions, between killing and letting die, is not itself morally relevant. Letting die constitutes 'the intentional termination of life' and therefore carries the same moral import.

Michael Tooley[26] also denies there is any difference of moral importance. If the motives, intentions, and other background factors are held constant and equal in both cases, there can be no moral difference. The main criticism of the doctrine is that there can be no justification for giving a doctor the right to withhold treatment, such as connecting a patient to a respirator, and yet to refuse him the right to withdraw treatment by disconnecting a patient already connected to the respirator.

The main reason the acts and omissions doctrine appears so inconsistent is because no distinction appears to be made between an omission in which something is *made to happen* and merely *letting something happen*. Such an argument could be used for claiming that a patient's disease caused his death, rather than the withdrawal of treatment. In cases of letting happen, the cause of death is Nature by way of the disease process. The doctor merely lets Nature take her course. It does not mean that the patient necessarily dies.

However, there are also cases of making happen. These are cases of omission. In the Rachels case described earlier, Jones has directly by his inaction not allowed any other outcome than the drowning. The question of whether some actual body movements occurred is irrelevant. What is important is whether 'making happen' occurred. Making a patient die by an omission is not no action at all and is open to the same extent of moral appraisal as killing the patient. Thus, when an omission occurs the omitter (the agent) has the intention, responsibility, and control of determining what will happen.

If turning off a ventilator (an inaction as we shall see) is such that every possible outcome is one in which the death of the patient must occur, then death has been brought about (i.e. made to happen). But if the turning off of a ventilator amounts only to making possible the death of the patient while at the same time leaving open other possible alternative outcomes for Nature or another agent to pursue, then merely 'letting die' is entailed.

Thus, under the normal situations pertaining to patients in the ICU, when ventilation is withdrawn the patient may, contrary to all expectations, breathe and many intensive care practioners can quote cases when this has happened to patients in their care. Once the patient has re-started breathing no attempt is made to stop this by drugs such as muscle relaxants. If the patient subsequently stops breathing and dies, then a letting die has occurred.

On the other hand, suppose that just prior to the ventilator withdrawal one is aware that not all the muscle relaxants given previously have worn off. Withdrawal of the ventilator at this time results in no possible outcome apart from the death of the patient. Making happen has therefore occurred because all possibilities of recovery have been denied.

Gillon believes that:[27]

Spurious philosophical claims or suggestions that when doctors forego life-prolonging treatment their omissions are necessarily morally equivalent to killing their patients must be rejected: in particular such ideas should not be allowed to bolster nonsensical notions that somehow doctors fall into the same moral camp as murderers unless they do all they possibly can to prolong their patients' lives, regardless of their patients' wishes, regardless of the costs and opportunity costs to others, regardless of the quality of life prolonged and regardless of the probabilities of achieving such prolongation. Such a result would indeed be a disastrous misinterpretation of the now uncontentious claim that there is no necessary moral difference between killing and letting die.

Gillon's use of the words 'letting die' is here equivalent to the 'making happen' described by the writer.

In an excellent article on guidelines for initiating and withdrawing life support Ruark and Raffin[24] acknowledge that once a treatment is started it is much more difficult to stop. Once a intravenous line is set up, it is difficult to then refrain from treating infections and disordered biochemistry. This is a form of 'slippery slope' in reverse. Once a treatment problem exists, it is much harder not to act. It may therefore be very difficult, for example, to withdraw renal dialysis, leading directly to the death of the patient.

The American Medical Association,[28,29] however, have accepted that there is no distinction between withholding and withdrawing life-sustaining treatment and this applies to all medical treatment which prolongs life, including nutrition and hydration. Fluid and nutrition, however, appear different to the writer. Patients in a persistent vegetative state or newborn babies cannot possibly feed themselves. Hence, withdrawing fluid and nutrition to my mind is a making happen because death is the only possible outcome. If doctors, moralists, and the law accept that this is permissible, they must also accept that this withdrawal endorses actively killing the patient.

In conclusion, there is no moral difference between killing and making die by an omission. What is morally true about acts causing deaths is equally true of omissions causing death, other things being equal.

It is claimed that it is simplistic to assume that a death that results from not connecting a patient to a respirator is morally preferable to a death that results from disconnecting a patient from a respirator.[27] However, in spite of the element of action in withdrawal of treatment, such as mechanical ventilation, it should be classified as a refusal to continue further treatment rather than an act of killing. An inaction occurs because it is the failure to re-start treatment that leads to the consequences. This shall be discussed further when the legal principles are examined.

On the other hand, it is claimed that there is a vital moral difference between withholding treatment with a view to causing death and withholding treatment because such treatment would be too burdensome to the patient, even though such an omission will lead to death, the crucial point being intention.[2] It is, however, very easy to say that a consequence was not intended but merely foreseen. This is the main criticism of the application of the doctrine to the withdrawal of food and nutrition.

Both the consequences of an action and the agent's beliefs and intentions about what he is doing are relevant to its moral assessment. This clearly leads on to the principle of 'double effect' in which Roman Catholic theologians claim that one can justifiably differentiate between those consequences of one's actions and inactions that are intended and those that are not intended, even though they may be foreseen.

5. Double effect

The main use of the principle of 'double effect' is to allow doctors to treat patients despite knowing that undesirable side-effects may arise out of that treatment. For example, the administration of pain-relieving drugs is allowed despite their use in doses that may coincidentally speed up death. It is claimed that:

In this case, of course, death is in no way intended or sought, even if the risk of it is reasonably taken; the intention is simply to relieve pain effectively, using for this purpose painkillers available in medicine.[30]

The principle therefore emphasizes the central moral importance of intentions, and elicits a sharp distinction between intended and foreseen (but unintended) consequences.[19,31] There can be consequences foreseen to be inevitable that do not count as intended means.[32]

The Appleton Consensus also states that pain and suffering should be vigorously treated, even if this leads to an earlier death.[15] The principle of double effect, although usually used in this setting of terminal pain relief, may also be used to justify the use of opiates in the relief of cough and breathlessness.[33] The principle, then, would appear to allow an agent to bring about indirectly a bad effect that it is not permissible to bring about directly.[19]

The Roman Catholic Church, as already mentioned, rejects the 'acts and omissions' doctrine, but it accepts the principle of 'double effect'.

There is a distinction between intending death and foreseeing that there is a serious risk of death as a result of one's act. The distinction is well understood and significant.[2]

However, not all cases of double effect are accepted by the Roman Catholic Church. When the dose of morphine is increased automatically at every administration or at daily intervals despite the patient not being in pain or distressed, this clearly is a case of active euthanasia, albeit by instalments.[2]

There are a number of arguments against the principle. For instance, one of the conditions for the principle to be valid is that the intention of any act must be solely to produce the good effect. The problem with this is that when one knows that a bad effect will result from one's action then it seems to be simply self-deceiving to say that one does not intend it.[34] It therefore encourages moral dishonesty.[31]

The principle further claims that a person does not intend all the consequences of an intentional action.[19] What counts as an intended effect is not, however, very clear. Intentions are difficult to define. How does one draw the line between intended means and foreseen inevitable consequences?[32] The term 'double effect' relates to side-effects which may be brought about in addition to the effect that is aimed at. A side-effect is claimed to be one not intended by the agent.[2] This cannot be correct, as the following example will show.

Consider an anaesthetic agent, the main effect of which is to send the patient to sleep. A side-effect is the production of hypotension. In a particular operation hypotension may be very desirable. Both drug A and drug B will anaesthetize the patient. Drug A, however causes, more hypotension (a side-effect) than drug B. Therefore in a particular operation requiring hypotension drug A is chosen. The side-effect here is surely intended. Similarly, consider an anaesthetic were no hypotension is required. If drug A is again used instead of B and the patient develops hypotension how can the anaesthetist deny responsibility by claiming it was only a foreseen consequence? What else did the anaesthetist expect?

Therefore, by far the greatest difficulty with the double effect principle is explaining how one does not necessarily intend a consequence that is foreseen. Almost anything can be foreseen as a side-effect rather than intended as a means. It would also be easy to say after an action that there was no intention to cause harm. If the agent was fully aware of the consequence before deciding to carry out the action, responsibility for that action must be accepted. The consequence of the action cannot be described as unintended, accidental, or indirect.

The double effect argument would therefore appear useful only to those holding absolutist principles[31] and reflects the moral absolutism of standard Roman Catholic morality. The following example clearly illustrates this. A Roman Catholic may not directly kill himself. However, if he is engaged in a just war he may throw himself on a grenade that lands in his foxhole to save his comrades. This is permissible as long as he does not intend to kill himself but only to absorb the shrapnel with his body, although he can surely foresee that this will lead to death. One effect it is claimed is intended (the absorbing of the shrapnel); the second effect (his death) is foreseen but not intended.[35] Many readers, I believe, would find it hard to accept there is a difference.

Does this mean that the principle of double effect is never acceptable? It appears that one of the few acceptable uses of the principle is in the context of terminal pain relief because one aspect that has not yet been mentioned is choice. No one would doubt that it is a moral imperative to prescribe pain killers for the relief of terminal pain. Not to do so would be one of the most immoral omissions in medicine. Therefore, there is no choice but to prescribe them. The doctor has no other option. The side-effects of the drugs are therefore irrelevant and hence, in this situation, the principle of double effect must be accepted.

6. Legal principles

The principles applied by the legal system are very much based on the ethical principles just discussed. For instance, specific court cases are beginning to expand the concept of best interests beyond the mere prolongation of life. Thus, in the past decade, statements such as the following have appeared in landmark court decisions:

The focal point of decision should be the prognosis as to the reasonable possibility of return to cognitive and sapient life, as distinguished from the forced continuance of that biological vegetative existence. . .[36]

'Prolongation of life' . . . does not mean a mere suspension of the act of dying, but contemplates at the very least, a remission of symptoms enabling return towards a normal, functioning, integrated existence.[37]

Courts in Britain have also recently started accepting that sometimes the quality of life of a person could be so bad that he or she should be allowed to die. These legal cases have mainly arisen in connection with decisions for further treatment of handicapped newborn babies.

In the case of in *Re B*[38] it had been accepted that there could be cases 'where the future was so certain and the life of the child was so bound to be full of pain and suffering' that the court might allow such a baby to die. Later, on 20 April 1989, the Appeal Court endorsed a High Court decision to allow a seriously handicapped baby, known as C, to die with as much comfort and dignity as possible.[39] Previously, in the High Court, Mr Justice Ward had held that baby C should be allowed to die because she had negligible if any intellectual function and since this was a hallmark of humanity any quality of life had already been denied to the child. Later, in November 1990, the Court of Appeal held that life-prolonging treatment could be withheld from another baby, known as J, because the Court believed the quality of his life was likely to be so poor that allowing him to die was in his best interests.[40]

In adult medicine, the principal judgment has been the Bland case,[41] in which it was stated that the sanctity of life principle was not absolute and, furthermore, existence in a persistent vegetative state was of no benefit to the patient.

Some may disagree with the notion that a person may be 'better off dead'. However, it is accepted that antibiotics are not administered to the terminally ill patient riddled with metastases. Not only is it futile but it would also be inhumane to keep life going to the bitter end. A quality of life judgement is made which accepts that the patient would be better off dead. In the case of baby J, the court approved the withholding of life-prolonging treatment, because after assessing the child's quality of life, it felt that such a life would be intolerable to him.[40]

The distinction between proportionate and disproportionate treatment is also supported in law. In *Barber* v. *Super Court*,[42] the Court held that:

Proportionate treatment is that which, in the view of the patient, has at least a reasonable chance of providing benefits to the patient which outweigh the burdens attendant to the treatment.

Life-sustaining treatment may be withheld or withdrawn . . . when . . . it is clear that the burdens of the patient's continued life with the treatment outweigh the benefits of that life for him. By this we mean that the patient is suffering, and will continue to suffer throughout the expected duration of his life, unavoidable pain, and that the net burdens of his prolonged life (the pain and suffering of his life with the treatment less the amount and duration of pain that the patient would likely experience if the treatment were withdrawn) markedly outweigh any physical pleasure, emotional enjoyment, or intellectual satisfaction that the patient may still be able to derive from life.[43]

A benefit thus exists when life-sustaining treatment contemplates

at the very least, a remission of symptoms enabling a return toward a normal functioning, integrated existence.[37]

With regard to the acts and omissions doctrine, the law of homicide in Britain appears to be quite clear. If a person acts and by that act hastens death, then that person could be charged with murder if the intention was to hasten death, or attempted murder if there was no such intention. If a person has a duty of care towards another, and omits to provide care such that death is hastened, then again that person could be charged with murder. If no duty of care exists, an omission is not legally recognized as a cause of death.

A crime can be committed by omission, but there can be no omission in law in the absence of a duty to act.[44]

Scottish law appears to go a step further in that one could be charged with 'wicked recklessness' by omission and be convicted of murder. However, once again, a duty of care between the murderer and the victim would have to be shown, otherwise the omission would not be legally recognized as the cause of death.

The law of homicide is equally applicable to doctors. Judge Devlin, in *R* v. *Adams*[45] stated that:

no doctor, nor any man, no more in the case of the dying than of the healthy, has the right deliberately to cut the thread of life.

Furthermore, in the case of *R* v. *Arthur*,[46] it was stated that

Doctors have no special powers to commit an act which causes death.

In this case the judge, in his direction to the jury, said:

. . . it is a very difficult area to decide precisely where a doctor is doing an act, a positive act, or allowing a course of events or a set of circumstances to ensue.

The courts attach great importance to the distinction because unless one has a duty to act, an omission does not lead to a legally recognized cause of death. On occasion, they have been faced with cases where a person who is charged with murder claims that it was not he who killed the victim but the hospital team who disconnected the life-support machine. In Britain the first of such cases appears to have been *Re Potter*.[47] In this case, the accused was committed for trial by the coroner on a charge of manslaughter. The assaulted victim had died from head injuries but his kidneys were removed for transplantation after ventilation had been commenced for that specific purpose. The accused raised a defence of *novus actus interveniens*, ascribing death to the donor operation. The prosecution was forced to charge assault only, for which the accused was duly convicted. It is interesting to note that no charges were brought against the medical staff. Subsequent decisions in the British courts have illustrated the rapid advances made in this field and similar claims have therefore been rejected.

In Scotland, in the seminal case of *Finlayson* v. *HM Advocate*[48] it was held that

once the initial reckless act causing injury has been committed, the natural consequence which the perpetrator must accept is that the victim's future depended on a number of circumstances, including whether any particular treatment was available and, if it was available, whether it was medically reasonable and justifiable to attempt it and to continue it.

Similarly, Lord Lane, in *R* v. *Malcherek* said[49]:

Whatever the strict logic of the matter may be, it is bizarre to suggest . . . that where a doctor tries his conscientious best to save the life of a patient . . . but fails in his attempt and therefore discontinues treatment (he) can be said to have caused the death of the patient.

Note, however, that he said 'whatever the strict logic may be'. Furthermore, neither judge actually defined what constituted death. In fact, Lord Lane stated:

Where a medical practitioner, using generally acceptable methods, came to the conclusion that the patient was *for all practical purposes dead* and that such vital functions as remained were being maintained solely by mechanical means, and accordingly discontinued treatment, that did not break the chain of causation between the initial injury and the death.

Thus, the fact that a doctor has commenced a particular course of life-prolonging treatment will not always oblige him to continue with it indefinitely, simply because it is prolonging the patient's life.[50]

The problem, from a legal point of view, is that stopping treatment, such as turning off a ventilator, could be seen as an act hastening death. The judgments in cases such as *R* v. *Malcherek*[49] and *R* v. *Cunningham*[51] indirectly did not contain any hint of criticism by the judges of the medical practice of withdrawing treatment from patients whom the judges believed to be still alive. According to Skegg,[50] there are two ways to avoid the conclusion that stopping treatment can be perceived by the law as an act causing death.

First, one could deny that the act of turning off the ventilator was for legal purposes a cause of death. Thus, Lord Devlin[52] has suggested that what would be regarded as good medical practice plays no part in legal causation. This is open to criticism.[50,53] It fudges the issues and appears to be 'playing with language'. It is also highly unlikely that the courts would accept as legal that a doctor could, by an act, kill the patient. This would set a very dangerous legal precedent. It is far more likely that the courts would manipulate the law concerning causation.[50]

Therefore, the second way would be to regard terminating ventilation as a 'letting happen' type of omission. If the doctor has no legal duty to provide care, then such an omission would not be regarded as a cause of death. Since a doctor is allowed to stop administering mouth-to-mouth resuscitation it could be argued that the ventilator is simply a form of mouth-to-mouth resuscitation and it could therefore be stopped.

Much the same reasoning was adopted in *Barber* v. *Superior Court*.[42] In this American case, the Appeal Court looked at the distinction between acts and omissions and concluded that the cessation of 'heroic' life-support measures was not an affirmative act but rather a withdrawal or omission of further treatment.

Even though these life support devices are, to a degree self-propelled, each pulsation of the respirator or each drop of fluid introduced into the patient's body by intravenous feeding devices is comparable to a manually administered injection or item of medication. Hence, disconnecting of the mechanical device is comparable to withholding the manually administered injection or medication.

The Court further held that there was no criminal liability for omissions unless there was a duty to act (similar to the law in Britain) and a doctor was under no duty to continue treatment once it had proved ineffective, thereby introducing the concept of futility and the distinction between proportionate and disproportionate treatment.

The doctor clearly acts when stopping the ventilator. However, it is not the stopping of the ventilator that leads to death but rather the failure to re-start it. If one could then argue that the doctor had no further duty of care, then the failure to start further treatment would not be seen from the legal stand-point to be the cause of death.

For example, the central argument in the Arthur case[46] was that, although it is not permissible for doctors to kill their patients, sometimes it is morally permissible to allow the patient to die. In this particular case, as the newborn infant had a severe handicap, it was permissible to let it die. The British Medical Association[54] rejects killing but is prepared to allow the withholding of life-saving treatment, even though that omission will lead to an earlier death than if treatment were given. In these cases, it is claimed, it is not the 'omitter' who is killing, but the disease or condition from which the patient suffers. An identical argument was used in the Bland case.[41]

However, as argued earlier, such a case is a 'making happen' and thus results in moral responsibility for the consequences arising out of the omission. Therefore, there appears to be a difference in the reasoning behind the ethical and legal principles. Ethically the distinction is based upon whether a 'making happen' or 'letting happen' occurs. The law appears to disregard this and instead stresses the importance of duty of care. However, in this writer's view, the duty of care test only applies to the distinction between proportionate and disproportionate treatment (there being no duty to provide disproportionate treatment). Therefore, despite the law's reliance on it, the duty of care test has no application in the acts and omissions doctrine.

Thus, in the Arthur case,[46] the correct order of reasoning was firstly to ascertain if a duty of care existed by examining whether the administration of nutrition to the child was ordinary (proportionate) or extraordinary (disproportionate) treatment. Having decided that treatment was extraordinary, no duty of care existed, and treatment could be withdrawn. It is essential to point out that a doctor looking after a particular patient may have a duty of care to administer treatment A (ordinary) but not treatment B (extraordinary). It is not an all or nothing phenomenon.

The problem from the legal standpoint is the obvious fact that withholding nutrition in a newborn must lead to death (the omission being a 'making happen') and therefore carries the equivalent moral responsibility as the deliberate act of killing the child. Since the courts cannot be seen to accept this they have fudged the whole issue by including duty of care within the acts and omissions doctrine.

There are, therefore, situations when turning off a ventilator would lead to a doctor being liable for murder. For example, if during the course of a routine operation in which the patient receives paralysing agents the anaesthetist turns off the ventilator, fully knowing the patient will die as a result, he is liable for murder. There is no doubt that the anaesthetist had a duty to care for the patient. This example adds weight to the consideration that withdrawal of ventilation is an inaction. Anaesthetists, during the course of operations, may, for a variety of perfectly acceptable medical reasons, stop ventilating the patient. It is the omission to re-start the ventilator, or at least, manual ventilation leading to the death of the patient that would attract ethical and legal repercussions and not the stopping of the ventilator *per se*. A duty of care exists and the omission to re-start treatment leads to the legal causation of death. In this situation, if the patient dies, it is clearly a case of 'making happen' and not one of 'letting die'.

The crucial test to ascertain whether a doctor has been in breach of his duty by failing to prolong a patient's life is whether in the same circumstances, a reasonable body of medical opinion would have managed the patient in the same way. Such an argument was also accepted in the Bland case.[41] Skegg[50] takes it a step further by claiming:

it is not enough that some reasonable doctors would have prolonged life: a doctor would not be convicted unless the jury accepts that in the circumstances *all* reasonable doctors would do so. [emphasis added]

Although this appears to be an extreme view, what is clear is that:

if a doctor terminated artificial ventilation in circumstances in which it could be regarded as good medical practice to do so, it is highly unlikely that he would be prosecuted for murder, or for any other criminal offence. It is even more unlikely that a jury would convict the doctor, whatever the judge said in the course of his summing-up.[50]

The principle of double effect also appears to be a fudge when examined from the legal standpoint. Kennedy, when discussing the options available in 'not prolonging dying', says that the 'double effect' policy has a blurring quality which makes prosecution less likely than in the case of an act with the unambiguous aim of speeding death.[32]

The case of *R* v. *Adams*[45] directly addressed the principle of double effect. Doctor Adams was charged with the murder of one of his patients by giving such large quantities of heroin and morphine that he must have known the drugs would kill her. Judge Devlin, in his address to the jury, said:

if the first purpose of medicine, the restoration of health, can no longer be achieved, there is still much for the doctor to do, and he is entitled to do all that is proper and necessary to relieve pain and suffering even if measures he takes may incidentally shorten life . . . the treatment was designed to promote comfort, and if it was the right and proper treatment, the fact that it shortened life did not convict him of murder.

It would therefore appear that Judge Devlin was accepting as correct the principle of double effect.

However, it is clear that if a doctor administers a drug that hastens death, he could be charged with murder, attempted murder, or manslaughter (culpable homicide in Scotland). Furthermore, as was decided in *R* v. *Hyam*[55] a person could be convicted of murder if he knew that it was 'highly probable' that death or grievous bodily harm would result from an act that he committed.

Glanville Williams states:[56]

there is no legal difference between desiring or intending a consequence as following from your conduct, and persisting in your conduct with a knowledge that the consequence will inevitably follow from it, though not desiring that consequence. When a result is foreseen as certain, it is the same as if it were desired or intended. It would be an undue refinement to distinguish between the two.

Therefore, it would appear that legally, what may be undesired may still be intended. This confirms the ethical arguments discussed earlier and indeed has been confirmed in recent legal cases.[57,58]

Although the law rarely distinguishes between intended and unintended though foreseen consequences, the courts sometimes manipulate the concept of causation, to avoid the conclusion that someone who foresaw that certain consequences would result from his act is necessarily legally responsible for them.[50] In other words, the acceptance in law of the principle of double effect does not rest on the 'no intention' point of view but instead would be based on 'no causation'. Thus, when morphine is used in high dosage in terminal pain relief, the cause of death is the disease rather that the drug.

On the other hand, Kennedy and Grubb[53] assert that the doctor by his act of administering such drugs intends the death of his patient and causes the death of the patient, but the intention is not culpable and the cause is not blameworthy because the law permits the doctor to do the act in question. While this will be disputed by many doctors (although accepted by many others), what is clear is that the law adopts the 'blind eye' approach[59] and allows such treatment because it cannot do otherwise. Society dictates that doctors who attend distressed terminally ill patients must be allowed to administer drugs, such as morphine (but not potassium), to produce relief. Administering these drugs must be regarded as the proper practice of medicine. Furthermore, it could certainly never be proven that an administered drug, given in reasonable dosage, caused the death of the patient. It is further argued that a reasonable dose in cases of patients with terminal illness is one which relieves pain.

The confusion in the law is highlighted by comments made by the Law Lords in the Bland case.[41] Lord Goff claimed that the drawing of a distinction between euthanasia and discontinuing treatment which leads to the death of the patient may lead to a charge of hypocrisy. Lord Lowry, in turn, introduced the concept of a distinction without a difference: the intention is to terminate life but the acceptable way of doing it is to discontinue a regime which the law has said that the doctors have no duty or even right to continue. Lord Browne-Wilkinson clearly believed that the conclusion reached would appear almost irrational. Finally Lord Mustill felt profound misgivings about the case and stated that however much the terminologies between euthanasia and withdrawing or withholding medical treatment may differ, the ethical status of the two courses of action were for all relevant purposes indistinguishable and the judgment in the case only served to emphasize the distortions of a legal structure which was already morally and intellectually misshapen.

From a purely philosophical standpoint, if one accepts that treatment, such as nutrition, can be withdrawn from a patient with the consequence that death will occur from starvation about two weeks later (with, it must be stressed no distress to the patient although the same cannot be said of the family or members of the health care team), surely one must also accept that it would be more morally justified to end such a life quickly by means of a lethal injection.

It is therefore difficult for this writer to accomodate the legal standpoint within the ethical principles discussed in this chapter. The law (which is only in place to serve society) should be founded on ethical reasoning. In such situations it is found wanting.

7. Conclusion

It is clear that the law accepts that assessments of quality of life are useful in certain situations. The law also accepts that doctors may give pain killers in acceptable doses at the end of life to relieve the distress of terminal disease, the legal basis for this being 'no causation' since causation cannot be proved. It has also been argued that the courts would allow the withdrawal of life-sustaining technology like artificial lung ventilation in certain situations, such as when no further duty of care is owed to the patient.

However, it must be accepted that the concepts of action and causation in relation to moral obligations are not entirely clear-cut and may even be paradoxical in places. Therefore, the dividing line between acts and omissions, between killing and letting die, between active and passive euthanasia is bound to be blurred at certain points.[60]

What is very clear is that, in caring for patients who are terminally ill the primary aim is no longer to extend life but to make the life that remains as comfortable and as meaningful as possible. A *Lancet* editorial,[61] although published under different circumstances, stressed that it would be unfortunate if the time came when no patient in hospital could decently die without a statutory period on the ventilator.

Treatments that are appropriate for acutely ill patients may be completely inappropriate for the dying. Cardiac resuscitation, artificial respiration, intravenous infusions, nasogastric tubes, and antibiotics are all primarily for use in acute (or acute on chronic) illnesses in order to assist the patient through a period of crisis towards recovery. Their use, without careful consideration of the intended purpose of that use, in the care of those approaching death is poor medical care.[2]

Notes

1. Angell M. (1990). Prisoners of technology. The case of Nancy Cruzan. *New England Journal of Medicine*, **322**, 1226–8.
2. Linacre Centre (1982). *Euthanasia and clinical practice: trends, principles and alternatives*. Working party. Linacre Centre, London.
3. Campbell, A.V. (1984). *Moral dilemmas in medicine*, (3rd edn). Churchill Livingstone, Edinburgh.
4. Pace, N., Plenderleith, J.L., and Dougall, J.R. (1991). Moral principles in withdrawing advanced life support. *British Journal of Hospital Medicine*, **45**, 169–70.
5. Smedira, N.G., *et al.* (1990). Withholding and withdrawal of life support from the critically ill. *New England Journal of Medicine*, **322**, 309–15.
6. Angell, M. (1982). The quality of mercy. *New England Journal of Medicine*, **306**, 98–9.
7. Schneiderman, L.J. and Spragg, R.G. (1988). Ethical decisions in discontinuing mechanical ventilation. *New England Journal of Medicine*, **318**, 984–8.
8. McCormick, R.A. (1974). To save or let die; the dilemma of modern medicine. *Journal of the American Medical Association*, **229**, 172–6.
9. Williams, A. (1988). Do we really need to measure the quality of life? *British Journal of Hospital Medicine*, **39**, 181.
10. Rachels, J. (1986). *The end of life*. Oxford University Press, Oxford.
11. Brazier, M. (1987). *Medicine, patients and the law*. Penguin, London.
12. Glover, J.G. (1990). The case of Ms Nancy Cruzan and the care of the elderly. *Journal of the American Geriatrics Society*, **38**, 588–93.
13. O'Donnell, T. (1957). *Morals in medicine*. Newman Press, Westminster, MD.
14. Dunstan, G.R. (1985). Hard questions in intensive care. *Anaesthesia*, **40**, 479–82.
15. Stanley, J. (1989). The Appleton Consensus: suggested international guidelines for decisions to forego medical treatment. *Journal of Medical Ethics*, **15**, 129–36.
16. Pius XII (1957). *Acta Apostolicae Sedis*, **49**, 1027–33.
17. Gillon, R. (1986). Ordinary and extraordinary means. *British Medical Journal*, **292**, 259–61.
18. Kelly, G. (1951). The duty to preserve life. *Theological Studies*, **12**, 550.
19. Beauchamp, T.L. and Childress, J.F. (1989). *Principles of biomedical ethics*, (3rd edn.) Oxford University Press, New York.

20. Jennett, B. (1991). Vegetative state: causes, management, ethical dilemmas. *Current Anaesthesia and Critical Care*, **2**, 57–61.

21. President's Commission (1983). *President's Commission for the Study of Ethical Problems in Medicine and Biomedical and Behavioural Research. Deciding to forego life-sustaining treatment: a report on the ethical, medical, and legal issues in treatment decisions.* Government Printing Office, Washington, DC.

22. Hastings Center (1987). *Guidelines on the termination of life sustaining treatment and the care of the dying.* Briarcliff Manor, The Hastings Center, New York.

23. AMA (American Medical Association) (1989). *Current opinions of the Council on Ethical and Judicial Affairs of the American Medical Association: Withholding or withdrawing life-prolonging treatment.* AMA, Chicago, Illinois.

24. Ruark, J.E. and Raffin, T.A. (1988). Initiating and withdrawing life support. Principles and practice in adult medicine. *New England Journal of Medicine*, **318**, 25–30.

25. Rachels J. (1975). Active and passive euthanasia. *New England Journal of Medicine*, **292**, 78–80.

26. Tooley, M. (1976). The termination of life: some issues. Manuscript, Research School of Social Sciences, Australian National University.

27. Gillon, R. (1988). Euthanasia, withholding life-prolonging treatment, and moral differences between killing and letting die. *Journal of Medical Ethics*, **14**, 115–17.

28. AMA (American Medical Association) (1986). AMA Council on Ethical and Judicial Affairs. Withholding or withdrawing life-prolonging medical treatment. *Journal of the American Medical Association*, **236**, 471.

29. AMA (American Medical Association) (1990). AMA Council on Scientific Affairs. Persistent Vegetative state and the decision to withdraw or withhold life support. *Journal of the American Medical Association*, **263**, 426–30.

30. Sacred Congregation for the Doctrine of the Faith, (1980). Declaration on Euthanasia. Vatican City. *Acta Apostolicae Sedis*, **72**, 542–52.

31. Downie, R.S. and Calman, K.C. (1987). *Healthy respect: ethics in health care.* Faber & Faber, London.

32. Kennedy, I. (1981). *The unmasking of medicine.* Allen & Unwin, London.

33. Dunstan, E.J. (1989). First know the patient: resolving multiple problems in old age. In *Doctors' decisions: Ethical conflicts in medical practice*, (ed. G.R. Dunstan and E.A. Shinebourne) pp. 187–96. Oxford University Press, Oxford.

34. Gillon, R. (1986). The principle of double effect and medical ethics. *British Medical Journal*, **292**, 193–4.

35. Engelhardt, H.T. (1986). *The foundations of bioethics.* Oxford University Press, New York:

36. Quinlan, (1976). 70 NJ 10, 355 A. 2d 647, cert. denied, 429 U.S. 922.

37. Dinnerstein Shirley (1978) Mass App 380 N.E. 2d 134.

38. *Re B* (1981). 1 WLR 421.

39. *Re C (a minor)*, [1989] All ER 782.

40. *Re J (a minor)*, [1990] 3 All ER 930.

41. *Airedale NHS Trust* v. *Bland* [1993] 2 WLR 316.

42. *Barber* v. *Los Angeles County Superior Court* (1983) 195 Cal Rptr. 484, 147 Cal.App. 3d 1006.

43. Conroy (1985) 98 NJ 321, 486 A.2d 1209.

44. Williams G, (1983). Textbook of criminal law, (2nd edn). Stevens & Sons, London.
45. *R* v. *Adams* (1957) Crim LR 365.
46. *R* v. *Arthur* (1981) *The Times*, 6 November.
47. *Re Potter* (1963) 31 *Medico-Legal Journal* 195.
48. *Finlayson* v. *HM Advocate* (1978) SLT (Notes) 60.
49. *R* v. *Malcherek* (1982) 2 All E.R. 422.
50. Skegg, P.D.G. (1984). *Law, ethics and medicine.* Clarendon Press, Oxford.
51. *R* v. *Cunningham* (1982) A.C. 566, 573.
52. Lord Devlin, P. (1962). *Samples of law making.* Oxford University Press, London.
53. Kennedy, I. and Grubb, A. (1989). *Medical Law: text and materials.* Butterworths, London.
54. BMA (British Medical Association) (1984). *Handbook of medical ethics.* British Medical Association, London.
55. *R* v. *Hyam* (1974) QB 99, (1975) AC 55.
56. Williams, G. (1958). *The sanctity of life and the criminal law.* Faber & Faber, London.
57. *R* v. *Maloney* (1985) AC 905.
58. *R* v. *Nedrick* (1986) 3 All ER 1.
59. Pace, N. (1991). Ethics of withdrawal of life-support. *Lancet*, 337, 495–6.
60. Walton, D.N. (1979). *On defining death.* McGill-Queen's University Press, Montreal.
61. Editorial (1974). Brain damage and brain death. *Lancet*, i, 341–2.

5

Advance directives: Legal and Ethical Considerations

Sheila A.M. McLean

The process of dying is deformed when it is subject to the violence of technological attenuation, drawn out and unduly extended by medical interventions, directly or indirectly. Technological brinkmanship is the most common way of creating the deformity . . .[1]

These rather stark words reflect a reality that irrespective of one's moral or religious beliefs, represents one reason why the issue of when and how one dies has come back to the forefront of debate in medical, legal, and ethical circles. They are also a sharp and forceful reminder that modern medical technology is not universally a good thing. There are several indications that those who feel themselves to be particularly vulnerable to the undesired application of life-sustaining therapy are choosing suicide rather than awaiting the moment's arrival.[2] Even without the use of invasive technology, there are conditions that individuals would choose to avoid and circumstances where they would prefer not to survive. Orentlicher,[3] for example, estimated that about 70 per cent of Americans will need to make a decision at some stage (or have one made for them) about whether or not to prolong therapy or to have it withheld or withdrawn.

This potential problem, therefore, affects a not insignificant group of the population. Of course, it also affects those who provide the therapy, not just in clinical, but also in human terms. In addition, the uncertainty of the current legal position further clouds the issue for those in the front line. There is a variety of situations where these problems—for patient and clinician—are combined. Should an apparently intended suicide attempt be treated? What is the legal standing of 'do not resusciate' (DNR) orders? When is treatment futile and therefore legitimately withheld, even against the wishes of patients or relatives?

Although these questions are complex, there is a potential legal answer to each of them, not least because, for the practitioner at least, there are clinical bases from which to explore the issues and reach a conclusion. However, this is very much less clear in other situations where the care decision is based not on whether or not it might work, but rather on the previously expressed wishes of the patient. Currently, it is widely accepted that the competent patient has an absolute right to refuse any and all treatment, even if it is life-enhancing or life-preserving. However frustrating for the health care provider, this is seen by the law as an inviolable exercise of patient autonomy that must be respected. Problems, however, arise where the patient is not competent, and recent cases in the UK and elsewhere have required resolution by law of whether or not an apparently competent refusal did indeed meet the law's standards of competency.

But what of the patient who is manifestly incompetent? Some conclusions about this situation were reached by the House of Lords in the Bland case,[4] and by the US Supreme Court in the Cruzan case.[5]

The Bland case concerned a young man who was injured in the Hillsborough disaster and had survived in a persistent vegetative state for some years thereafter. His family and care team agreed that, since his condition was irreversible, it would be better if artifical feeding could be stopped in order that he might die. The House of Lords endorsed this decision, declaring it not to be unlawful in this case for nutrition and hydration to be stopped. In the Cruzan case, the court demanded 'clear and convincing' evidence that the young woman in question, who was also in a persistent vegetative state, would have chosen not to survive in that condition before authorizing removal of treatment which could prolong her life.

The conclusions reached in these cases referred to a particular group of people in a specific set of circumstances. The apparent fear of being disenfranchised at the end of life has, however, generated a new group of patients: those who wish, *in advance of incompetence*, to have the final say in whether or not they should be kept alive. Thus, increasingly, there is an interest in the making of what are variously called durable powers of attorney, advance directives, or 'living wills'. For the purposes of this chapter, the form 'advance directive' is preferred, not least because the term 'living will' might confuse the issue. What is *not* being made is a declaration on a par with the kind of will made in exercise of the individual's testamentary capacity. There is no right of ownership in the human body that makes its post-mortem disposal as simple as that of property, and, in any event, it is clear that the actuation of the advance directive occurs *before* and *not after* death, and its consequences are infinitely more grave than the mere disposal of money and household goods.

1. Why make an advance directive?

Without doubt, some people fear the inappropriate use of technology when their death is imminent or the process of dying can be prolonged. However miraculous the capacities of modern medicine, its means may be seen by some as degrading, diminishing, and unacceptable. For these people, the capacity to control, while control is still possible, whether or not they will be maintained in this situation is an essential part of respect for their own autonomy. Or as Kuczewski[6] puts it, '. . . the living will expresses the values by which one lives and is committed to living. It encodes the desire for treatment and a death in accordance with one's commitment to these values . . . the living will is an expression of the good in accordance with which one lives his or her life'.[7] These words reflect more than mere symbolism. The value for the individual patient in the making of an advance directive is also the expectation that clinicians will pay attention to its terms, that it provides for currently competent individuals '. . . certainty and assurance about how they will be treated when incompetent, thus serving the interests of competent patients in controlling their future'.[8] This reassurance, which is an integral part of the desire to make a declaration about future health care decisions, is vitally dependent, therefore, on the validity of the instrument itself. If it is not legally endorsed and clinically observed, its main purpose evaporates.

Two issues arise here. The first is whether or not the nature of the document itself makes it worthy of legal or medical respect, and the second relates to what approach is actually taken by the law. Each of these will be considered in turn.

2. Do advance directives merit respect?

Given the significance of the outcome predicated by following an advance directive, many are acutely concerned about the extent to which competent individuals can possibly make a definitive statement about what should happen to them when they are no longer competent. Two main strands of concern emerge.

The first relates to whether or not we can really know that the individual still holds to the beliefs and still feels the concerns which provoked the making of the directive in the first place. For some commentators, this should be taken as definitive of the status to be given to advance directive. They would argue that to make an automatic assumption that the same interests prevail after the fact of illness and incompetence disvalues the incompetent. As Robertson, for example, says, '. . . the prior directive is taken to be the most accurate indicator of the person's interests once she becomes incompetent. The problem, however, is that the patient's interests when incompetent—viewed from her current perspective—are no longer informed by the interests and values she had when competent'.[8]

To turn Robertson's argument around, however, we equally do not know that the person does *not* continue to share precisely the same sets of beliefs, and hold the same set of interests, that were held before incompetence. Absent evidence of this, it arguably disvalues the competent to presume that things will have changed. It atomizes their life rather than seeing it as part of a continuum of values. Of course, if one held Robertson's view, and since there is no way of knowing whether or not these views *have* changed, the logical outcome is that the previously expressed wishes of the patient would have to be ignored unless they fit the preferred clinical treatment. This may not inevitably be problematic, of course. In a survey of 126 competent residents of a nursing home and 49 family members over a period of two years, Danis *et al.*[9] concluded that the treatment given to patients when incompetent accorded with their advance directives in 75 per cent of cases. Thus, most of the time doctors' decisions were in accord with what their patients would have wanted, but not always. In fact, this same study found that: '[T]he presence of the written advance directive in the medical record did not facilitate this consistency . . .'[10] In other words, the patient's advance decision merely accorded with what doctors believed to be the correct medical outcome.

Quite apart from the question of respect, which for proponents of advance directives is the central value here, paradoxically this conclusion goes some way towards defeating the second main reason for opposing respecting them. There are, according to some commentators, . . . intrinsic limitations to giving prior instructions. Patients may find it difficult to understand all the relevant medical issues . . .'[11] However, it would appear that the majority of patients in the sample referred to above reached (in advance) the same conclusion as their doctor. That this is so, somewhat minimizes the argument of the inability to understand. However, these same authors also point to a further problem that equally requires resolution.

In making an advance directive, a decision has to be made about whether or not it should cover only specific future circumstances or should be general. The difficulties of interpreting a general statement are obvious and need not be discussed, but even when specific conditions are referred to in the directive, '. . . the clinical circumstances may be different from what the patient anticipated, making it necessary to adapt the patient's explicitly stated preferences to the actual situation'.[11] Now, if one were only taking about a distaste for a particular therapy, this objection would have considerable weight. However, surely the patient is doing something quite different, no matter how hard it may be for some to accept. The patient is expressing a wish not to continue to live in *circumstances* or *conditions*, which for them are unacceptable. It may not matter what the form of medical intervention takes, but it does matter that their lives are restricted by mental and physical limitations—whatever their cause and whatever could be done by way of palliation. Arguably, it is this which is vital, rather than whether or not the specific condition was envisaged. The individual's concern is about *quality* of life, nor the *clinical* condition.

Certainly, no one could dispute that an unequivocal advance directive, which offers those who act on it and those who care for the patient the reassurance that they are acting for the best, could be achieved, However, its effect would necessarily be limited unless one concedes the point just made concerning quality of life. But the clarity of the declaration is only one issue on whether or not it is respected. Vindication of expressed wishes depends on those who carry it out actually endorsing it when the reality of the illness confronts them. By definition, all acts pursuant to an advance directive's terms are carried out by proxy. Given that they are not in the incompetent patient's position, alternative decision-makers can have no certain knowledge of what the individual currently feels, and will themselves usually have a preference for life over death. Human nature would, presumably, make them cautious and conservative about participating in an event that is inimical to *their* present understanding and desires. Evidence that this is the case is supported by research concerning proxy decision-makers' attitudes.

The use of proxies is particularly relevant to the so-called durable power of attorney, but is feasible in any form of advance directive. L.L. Emanuel and E.J. Emanuel[11] suggest that, '[f]or a proxy to carry out the patient's wishes, several things must happen. First, patients must designate a proxy. Then they must discuss their treatment preferences with the proxy. Next, the proxy must understand the patient's preferences, and finally, the proxy must make the same choices as the patient would have'.[12] However, the reality is not as straight forward. For example, they found when that even when proxies were nominated, only between 16 and 55 per cent of patients actually discussed their preferences in advance. Moreover, proxies were more reluctant to authorize discontinuation of life-sustaining treatment than the patients themselves were. The authors concluded that, '. . . at best, proxies will accurately reflect the wishes regarding life-sustaining treatment of about 68 per cent of the patients who have appointed them . . . Moreover, of the proxies who do manage accurately to judge patients' wishes, less than two-thirds will be emotionally capable of carrying them out.'[13] Perhaps for these reasons, the House of Lords Select Committee on Medical Ethics stated, whilst recognizing arguments in favour of proxy decision-making, that; '. . . we do not favour the more widespread development of such a system'.[14] However, it should be borne in mind that this recommendation merely relates to the formal naming of a specific individual to whom certain powers are given. It would be naïve to think that this comment goes beyond this. Where no named proxy has been elected, this does not mean that decisions are not actually taken by proxy. Either the doctor him or herself will reach a conclusion (unless the advance directive is binding on them) or they will routinely consult relatives, even although where the patient is an adult it is generally the case that nobody else—not even a close relative—can legally provide or withhold consent on their behalf. In other words, in the absence of binding advance directives, decisions are always taken by proxy, even when they happen to coincide with the advance wishes of the patient. It is a matter of some surprise, therefore, that the Select Committee (and many others) have devoted such energy to this question of proxy decision making.

Even, if we accept the narrower description of the proxy decision that is routinely applied, and if named proxies are not to be encouraged, we are still confronted with the original concept of the advance directive, namely, that it expresses the competent person's predictive exercise of autonomy. Whatever form such directives take, even opponents will generally concede that this is the aim of the document, whether or not they believe that it can actually be trusted to achieve it.

3. The legal view: a comparative analysis

Before considering current British law on advance directives, it is worth making a brief foray into other jurisdictions. In some countries, the system of advance directives has a long pedigree and the benefits and drawbacks of legal endorsement have been investigated in more detail. Although British law has, until recently, maintained a virtual silence on this topic, other countries have attempted to grasp the nettle. This, perhaps unsurprisingly, is particularly so in the US, although other countries, such as Denmark, have recently drafted legislation for advance directives.[15]

In America, virtually every state and the District of Columbia now have laws covering advance directives.[16] This widespread legal commitment was further recognized in the Patient Self-Determination Act 1990 which, broadly speaking, requires all federal or medicaid-funded care givers to notify their patients of the state law on advance directives and of their right to make one. This law was intended to bring state policy to public attention, although it does not in itself give patients any new rights.[17] There was obviously a perception that the advance directive could fulfil a positive function—most likely the endorsement of autonomy—or at least that the spirit of the law could encourage the public to consider making advance directives.

As suggested earlier, it is not surprising that the US is leading developments in this area, and the reason for this is evident. Few countries pay such legal and/or symbolic attention to the concept of autonomy as the US. From the early decision in *Schloendorff*[18] and the development of the so-called privacy right from cases such as *Skinner* v. *Oklahoma*[19] and *Roe* v. *Wade*[20] and against the backdrop of a constitutional bill of rights, a central tenet of the resolution of conflict between the individual and the State (or other groups) has been the right of competent persons to make decisions about what happens to themselves, subject only to clearly deprived and limited circumstances.

If the advance directive is an extension of the right to self-determination (to act autonomously), then there are few juristic cultures more apparently amendable to its development and endorsement than the US. This is not to say that implementation is not without problems, however. Debate, both practical and academic, rather than consensus, continues to characterize the approach to the directives, their inherent value and ultimate efficacy. Some attention is now paid to this question.

Although the number of people taking advantage of the law is not an unassailable test of its efficacy, there are some interesting data from US research (see below). Certainly, there is emotional, moral, and clinical controversy over whether or not advance directives should exist or be respected. However, a possible solution might be to consider whether advance directives fulfil a need that is greater than any arguments against them. If a directive serves the purpose of reassuring people that their wishes will be respected, that their right to autonomy does not cease with their lapse into incompetence, and if these are matters of vital importance to the individual, then one might expect two consequences. First, that the take-up rate would be high, and secondly, that the terms of the advance directives would be respected. Evidence from the US, however, does not support either of these expectations. Although in Denmark substantial numbers of eligible citizens have made advance directives,[21] evidence from the US, where this has been an option for much longer, is equivocal. The Emanuels,[11] for example, estimate that even after the *Cruzan* case, which demonstrated the problems of not having made an advance directive, only about 20 per cent of patients took advantage of their right to make such a directive.[22] This figure admittedly represented an increase, presumably in part due to the widespread media coverage of this case, because two years earlier, Emanuel *et al.*[16] noted that: '. . . advance directives are infrequently used. In 1987 only 9 per cent of Americans had written advance directives for medical were care . . .'[23] If the value of legal endorsement of advance directives were measured by this alone, it might be thought that the emotion and moral concern generated by them is scarcely worth the effort. Where a 'right' is supremely contentious (indeed, offensive to some) might it not be defeasible to the arguments against it if nobody wants to exercise it anyway?

Even if this were a legitimate perspective, however, further evidence would suggest that to use the number of directives actually made as a yardstick of whether or not people wanted them would be a serious mistake. People's attitudes to the end of life cannot exclusively be drawn from whether or not they make a formal declaration in advance. For example, it was reported that a Harvard University/*Boston Globe* poll carried out in 1991 indicated that two-thirds of respondents favoured doctor-assisted suicide and euthanasia on request by a terminally ill patient.[24] Further, Emanuel *et al.*[25] found that 93 per cent of their sample indicated that they favoured some form of planning for the end of their lives, although few had made any arrangements. As they report: '[A]lthough 57 per cent of the patients wanted a document specifying future care, only 7 per cent had one; and although 59 per cent wanted a discussion with their physicians, only 5 per cent reported having had such a discussion . . .'[25] As in the case of organ donor cards, the interest in planning is there, even if it is not always formalized. Although by no means a definitive argument in favour of advance directives, these data suggest that the right to make one is highly valued.

The second expectation (i.e. that advance directives would be respected) has also not been supported by research. In part, this is because directives are not always known about (again in analogy with organ donor cards). This is a problem that some believe could be resolved by centralized documentation of their existence. In Denmark, for example:

If a patient is in a situation covered by a living-will form, and if he is unable to exercise his right of self-determination, the physician who is treating the patient shall be required to examine the Living-Will Register in order to find out whether the patient has expressed any wishes therein in connection with his treatment.[26]

However, recent evidence from Denmark suggests that even this mechanism may not be completely successful. It has been reported that: 'Some 45 000 people have made a "living will" since the legislation came into force . . . out of a total population of 5.1 million . . . but only one or two doctors are consulting the computerized register each week'.[21] Although the law is relatively recent it will be instructive to know whether or not awareness of advance directives is ultimately enhanced by the maintenance of a central register. In America, where no central register is maintained, the Emanuels reported that 'of all the advance directives that were completed, only 31 per cent were available when life-sustaining treatment decisions were being made . . .'[12]

Again, concerning the efficacy of the advance directive, the Emanuels report that, '22.8 per cent were ignored or overridden even when they were available'.[12] Here, of course, the concept of commitment to patient self-determination comes up against the clinical perception of what is best for the patient. In addition, doubts about whether or not the circumstances currently in existence are the same as those contemplated by the patient when drafting the directive will also be likely to influence the decision-maker. Just as other proxies (e.g. relatives) are more likely to opt for continuation of treatment, so too are doctors, who are third party proxies in these circumstances. Obviously, it is distressing for the doctor to have to endorse a competent patient's wish for a hastier death, especially when therapy is available that might prolong life. However, it is probably even more distressing, in the case of an incompetent patient, when the doctor shares some of the doubts identified earlier concerning whether or not the patient would now still wish to adhere to previously expressed wishes.

This very scenario recently confronted a Canadian doctor and it is instructive to evaluate briefly the attitude of the court. In the case of *Malette* v. *Shulman et al.*[27] Mrs Malette sued Dr Shulman for assault. The victim of a serious road traffic accident, Mrs Malette was brought into hospital, where it was finally concluded that she required a blood transfusion if her life were to be saved. Mrs Malette was a Jehovah's witness and carried a card indicating that she would not wish to receive blood transfusion under any circumstances. The card made it clear that she was aware of the consequences of her decision but insisted that no transfusion should be given, even to preserve her life. Dr Shulman was aware of the existence of this card, but overrode its terms with the aim of saving her life. The court found in favour of Mrs Malette, saying, '[a] doctor is not free to disregard a patient's advance instructions any more than he would be free to disregard instructions given at the time of the emergency'.[28]

Although, somewhat oddly, denying that this case concerned advance directives (apparently on the basis that such terminology was only appropriate where the patient was expressing an actual desire to die), arguably this is precisely what the court was considering. Certainly, one point was made absolutely clear: 'Regardless of the doctor's opinion, it is the patient who has the final say on whether to undergo the treatment'.[29] Whatever terminology one applies to the law's approach, however, the issue of compliance is clearly of central importance. Perhaps for this reason, Danish law is extremely clear on this point: 'The testator's wishes . . . shall be binding for the attending physician'.[30]

4. The UK position

Despite the efforts of numerous pressure groups, and considerable debate, until recently the standing of advance directives was uncertain. However, recent cases, culminating in the report of the House of Lords Select Committee on Medical Ethics,[14] have offered some clarification. An evaluation of current law now follows.

One point should, however, be made at the outset. Even if relatively underused, even unsuccessful, the development of laws concerning advance directives in other jurisdictions was, as has already been pointed out, predicated on a notion of patient autonomy enshrined in case law and/or constitution. It would be a gross exaggeration to suggest that law-makers in Britain have shown such an unequivocal commitment to this philosophy. Decisions concerning patient care are routinely subject to a professional-centered rather than a patient-centred analysis.[31] The jurisprudence of patient autonomy has been at best badly developed and at worst absent. Even the competent patient who refuses life-saving treatment, despite the use of rhetoric which mimics that of the US courts, may find his or her expressed refusal overridden in some situations.[32]

Recently, however, a certain shift has become apparent. For example, in the 1992 case of *Re T*,[33] it was indicated that when an informed and competent patient makes an anticipatory choice which is clearly expressed and applies to the circumstances in question, a doctor would be bound to follow it. In this case, the court believed that the young woman in question, who was refusing a blood transfusion, was not acting freely and therefore did not recognize her decision as being competent. Perhaps, however, it was the Bland case,[4] which reached the House of Lords in 1993, which finally forced Britain's legal community to address these issues head on. Although the Bland case concerned a patient in a persistent vegetative state (PVS), and who had not written an advance directive, the distressing and far-reaching implications of this case were not lost on the public or the judiciary. Indeed, in this case, although not directly required to comment on this point, Lord Goff took the opportunity of making the following statement:

It has been held that a patient of sound mind may, if properly informed, require that life support should be discontinued . . . the same principle applies where the patient's refusal to give his consent has been expressed at an earlier date, before he became unconscious or otherwise incapable of communicating it.[34]

Although implying that an advance directive was legally valid in the UK, this remark could not establish a precedent. However, it did give rise to the hope that the law might change. The British Medical Association (BMA) had endorsed the value of advance directives in a statement in 1992 and did so again, more forcefully, in 1994.[35] The Medical Treatment (Advance Directives) Bill was introduced into the House of Lords in the 1992–3 session. Although this Bill did not require doctors to follow the terms of a directive, it sought to clarify that no criminal offence would be committed by a doctor who did comply with it. A Consultation Paper produced by the Law Commission in 1993 went further, declaring that a refusal of treatment made in advance should carry as much weight as a refusal by a currently competent patient.[36] In *Re C*,[37] the Family Division of the High Court indicated that it was 'common ground that a refusal can take the form of a declaration of intention never to consent in the future or never to consent in some future circumstances'.[38] In the meantime, the Declaration of the Standing Committee of Doctors of the EC on Living Wills/Advance Directives (1993) stated that, '[i]n the absence of contrary evidence, a valid statement of wish and intention is of value in representing a patient's settled wish when the patient may no longer be competent to express a view.'[39]

Thus, this recent flurry of legal activity has gone some way to validating the status of the advance directive as some form of legally important document. However, despite what can clearly be seen as a move towards recognizing the power of a directive on health care choices, the law has remained ultimately uncertain. Most particularly, what was uncertain—and what, as has been said already, is critical to the standing of such directives—was the extent to which the directive should be respected by the doctor. It is one thing to say that people are at liberty to *make* such a statement, and quite another to indicate that it will be carried out, and it was this issue that many hoped the House of Lords Select Committee would resolve.

In a sense, the Select Committee achieved this, but in a manner that can be criticized as being unsatisfactory, at least from the perspective of those who see the ultimate value being protected as being the autonomy of the individual. Given the conflicting evidence about the standing of the advance directive, some felt that the only way to resolve this was by way of legislation, perhaps similar to the Danish model. Certainly, the somewhat half-hearted US approach might suggest that—unusually, perhaps, in matters of this sensitivity and complexity—forceful legislation could be a desirable option. Interestingly, despite previous resistance to legislation, the BMA's 1994 Statement approved limited legislation to clarify the non-liability of the doctor who acts in accordance with such a directive.[40]

However, like their counterparts in the European Union, the BMA was not in favour of advance directives being in all circumstances binding on the doctor. Undoubtedly the same considerations that have acted to limit their unchallenged implementation in other countries also had some influence on the BMA. Nonetheless, the fear that declarations made in advance may no longer accurately reflect the current wishes of the patient is only one characteristic of this conclusion. In a legal system, which often seems to prefer the clinical to the personal decision, the matter under debate is medicalized to the extent that the choice becomes medical rather than personal. However, the Select Committee clarified that advance directives have *some* legal standing, even if they were not prepared to go any further. The Committee felt that it was unnecessary to legislate for advance directives since the ethical commitment to honouring them was increasingly being recognized by doctors and case law. The clinching point, however, was that, '. . . it could well be impossible to give advance directives in general greater legal force without depriving patients of the benefit of the doctor's professional expertise and of new treatments and procedures which may have become available since the advance directive was signed'.[41] Their conclusion was that this matter was best dealt with by the drafting (by representatives of the medical professions) of a code of practice, although the

. . . informing premise of the code should be that advance directives must be respected as an authoritative statement of the patient's wishes in respect of treatment. Those wishes should be overruled only where there are reasonable grounds to believe that the clinical circumstances which actually prevail are significantly different from those which the patient had anticipated, or that the patient had changed his or her views since the directive was prepared . . .[42]

This conclusion is of arguable logic. The patient will have expressed in advance the conditions that he or she finds intolerable to contemplate, and therefore no other condition could trigger consideration of an advance directive. Unless we are obsessed with clinical terminology, such conditions can be described in human terms; they reflect a *quality* of existence and not a *clinical* condition. Also, if there is any reason to believe that the patient has changed his or her mind, and this would always have to be tested, then again the advance directive's instructions are not triggered since it is no longer representative of the patient's wishes. To the present author, these counter-arguments seem to suggest that the real reasons for not wishing to render advance directives always binding was more about not wishing to interfere with clinical freedom than about concern regarding the contemporary validity of the directive itself.

So where does this leave the patient who seeks the reassurance that they can anticipate the unthinkable, and have their anticipatory choice vindicated? Little, if any, attention was paid by the Select Committee to the lessons learned from other, more experienced, legal systems. Some of their concerns might, for example, have been allayed by concentration on the *form* of the directive rather than its mere existence. Perhaps a specific rather than a general form might have eased some of their fears, even if, as argued above, this misses the point. Or, the model developed by the Seattle Veterans Affairs Medical Center might have been addressed. This model uses a values history in an attempt to minimize any incongruence between past and (potential) present wishes. By viewing the patient as a whole person with values which are central to their preferences (as opposed to transient and temporal) this form seeks to reduce any potential for the 'wrong' decision to be taken whilst at the same time reinforcing the underlying autonomy values which give advance directives their standing in the first place.[43]

The Select Committee's recommendations will not reassure those who fear unwanted medical prolongation of life. Neither will they help those whose wishes may be sought to fulfil the desires of their loved ones. In all, then, this Report makes very little headway, and contains few surprises. At best, what it establishes is that doctors will not be liable if they act in accordance with a competently executed directive, but—although important—this was scarcely the central issue. Indeed, their conclusions fit rather well with the views of Robertson, a partial sceptic about advance directives, who concludes:

Rather than simply enforce all prior directives, doctors, family, and others involved in the care of incompetent patients should be able to question whether the patient's interests would be best served by actions contrary to the living will, in situations in which the incompetent patient appears to have an interest in further life.[44]

In other words, even though an individual may have made an unequivocal statement about preferences, this can be ignored if it 'appears' (to someone else) that the person may have been wrong, or may now be wrong. We do not generally do this with the competent patient, so why, it may be asked, should this be permissible with the patient who competently expressed the same wish—the only difference, after all, is temporal, it is not based on principle.

5. Conclusion

The current position is unsatisfactory. In fact, it has the peculiarity of being of little value to the patient, the doctor, and the law. What can be done? One suggestion raised above is that forceful legislation could be introduced, but this would only resolve the situation if it were in indisputable terms.

The law could, of course, render advance directives utterly meaningless and without legal standing. This would certainly solve the interpretational problems, but it would also sit ill with legal and social trends. If, on the other hand, the law were to be changed towards respecting advance directives it would have required to make an outright commitment to honouring them. Otherwise it would not have changed the law at all and would have been redundant. There is, of course occasional symbolic value in legislation, such as the US 1990 Patient Self-Determination Act, but its effect seems to be minimal in matters of this sort. The good take-up of the advance directive in Denmark could be explained not by the fact that the law exists only as a theoretical device, but rather by the unequivocal commitment to respecting the directive once made.

However, for many reasons, a law which rendered advance directives binding in all circumstances would probably have been unpopular and may even have been unworkable in the UK. But it would have been necessary if our current, somewhat cloudy, legal position were to progress towards respect for the competently expressed choices of the potential incompetent. Evidence shows that where the laws concerning advance directives are equivocal, the law itself becomes of secondary importance. Stevens and Hassan,[45] for example, reporting on a survey of medical practitioners in South Australia, where patient self-determination legislation is in place, reached a critical conclusion:

The findings . . . indicate that higher proportions of respondents used internalised ethical and moral values to guide their decision-making than the proportion who depended on externally imposed legal sanctions to circumscribe their actions. These and previous findings suggest, first, that alteration or clarification of the law would not necessarily change the practices of individual medical practitioners, and second, that questions of legality are currently not the principal considerations used when making decisions to withhold or withdraw treatment or to terminate the lives of patients.[46]

Others have objected that enshrining a right to choose death in our law represents a breakdown of civilized values. Mayo,[47] for example, says, '[t]he history of our activities and beliefs concerning the ethics of death and dying is a history of lost distinctions of former significance'.[48]

Whatever the conclusion on these matters, it appears that legislation may not yet be the appropriate vehicle to synthesize strongly held opposing views, on a matter of such fundamental importance, unless it is prepared to be definitive one way or the other. Currently, British law merely relieves the physician of liability when acting in good faith. It has shown itself unwilling, or unable, to address the claims of potential patients for a direct and respected say in their own medical management at the end of their lives.

Perhaps, then, the answer does not lie in legislating for or against advance directives but in re-evaluating our commitment to individual autonomy, and the values to which we claim to subscribe. In the West, at least, autonomy individualizes, but need not fragment, communities. Moving to legislate decisively in favour of advance directives may be an ultimate goal, but more must be known about them. Even in the US, commentators lament the lack of research that could help to solve this dilemma. Lynn and Teno,[49] for example, suggest that, '[w]hile the theoretical justifications for the use of advance directives are easy to marshall, to date little empirical research has been done to assess the merits of advance directives in practice'. They continue,

... advance directives have been proposed as the answer to the problem of how to empower patients so that they maintain control of their care even when incompetent. We have not yet shown that directives will answer that need. Indeed, the question may well be better articulated as one of defining and implementing an optimal procedure to make care decisions on behalf of incompetent adults. We certainly do not know how well advance directives answer that need, especially in comparison to alternative strategies. We may have the wrong answer; in fact, we may have answered the wrong question.[50]

What seems clear is that until these issues can be resolved, it may well be premature to seek directive legislative intervention. However, it must also be borne in mind that—assuming such clarity is, or can be, achieved—it will be to the law that we must ultimately look for encapsulation of the value systems that emerge. If respect for anticipatory decisions is to be a part of our culture, we would do well to bear in mind the words of one commentator:

The law is about human beings. And the law governing the termination of life-sustaining treatment is a particularly human matter—how people come to their death, and how we treat those nearing the end. It is about choosing between a society that honors our preferences, embeddedness in relationships, and control of our bodies, or a society that leaves us stranded, defenseless, and imprisoned at the end.[51]

Notes

1. Callahan, D. (1993). Pursuing a peaceful death. *Hastings Center Report*, 23, 34.
2. Kamisar, Y. (1993). Are laws against assisted suicide unconstitutional? *Hastings Center Report*, 23, 32. See also p. 38, 'Suicides by people over the age of sixty account for about 25 percent of all suicides'.
3. Ohrentlicher, D. (1991). Advance medical directives. *Journal of the American Medical Association*, 260, 410. See also Young, E.W.D. and Jex, S.A. (1992). The patient self-determination act: potential ethical quandaries and benefits'. *Cambridge Quarterly of Healthcare Ethics*, 1, 107.
4. *Airedale NHS Trust* v. *Bland* [1993] 1 All ER 821.
5. *Cruzan* v. *Director, Missouri Dept. of Health* (1990) 110 S.Ct. 2841.
6. Kuczewski, M.G. (1994). Whose will is it, anyway? A discussion of advance directives, personal identity and consensus in medical ethics. *Bioethics*, 8, 27.
7. Note 6, p. 35.
8. Robertson, J. (1991). Second thoughts on living wills. *Hastings Center Report*, 6, 7.
9. Danis, M. *et al.*, (1991). A prospective study of advance directives for life-sustaining Care. *New England Journal of Medicine*, 324, 884.
10. Note 9, p. 885.

11. Emanuel, L.L. and Emanuel, E.J. (1963). Decisions at the end of life: guided by communities of patients. *Hastings Center Report*, **23**, p. 6.
12. Note 11, p. 7.
13. Note 11, p. 8.
14. House of Lords (1994). *Report of the Select Committee on Medical Ethics*. Vol. I: Report, p. 56, para. 271. HL Paper 21.1. HMSO, London.
15. Order No. 782 of 18 September 1992.
16. Emanuel L.L., *et al.* (1991). Advance directives for medical care—a case for greater use. *New England Journal of Medicine*, **324**, 880.
17. Capron, A.M. (1992). The Patient Self-determination Act: a cooperative model for implementation. *Cambridge Quarterly of Healthcare Ethics*, **1**, 97.
18. *Schloendorff* v. *Society of New York Hospital* 105 NE 92 (NY, 1914).
19. *Skinner* v. *Oklahoma* 316 U.S. 535 (1942).
20. *Roe* v. *Wade* 93 S.Ct. 705 (1973).
21. Dolley, M. (1993). Public uses Denmark's living will. *British Medical Journal*, **306**, 414.
22. Note 11, p. 7.
23. Note 16, p. 889.
24. Smith II, G.P. (1993). Reviving the swan, extending the curse of Methusela, or adhering to the Kevorkian ethics?. *Cambridge Quarterly of Healthcare Ethics*, **2**, 50.
25. Note 16, p. 891: 'Despite the large proportion of respondents who said they desired some form of planning, few had actually made explicit arrangements before the interview'.
26. Note 15, s.4.
27. *Malette* v. *Shulman et al.* [1991] 2 Med LR 162.
28. Note 27, p. 165.
29. Per Robins, J.A., p. 164.
30. Note 15, s.3(2).
31. McLean, S.A.M. (1989). *A patient's right to know: information disclosure, the doctor and the law*. Dartmouth, Aldershot.
32. cf. *Re S* (Adult: Refusal of treatment) [1992] 3 WLR 806.
33. *Re T* [1992] 4 All ER 649
34. Note 4, p. 866.
35. BMA Statement on Advance Directives, January 1994, p. 1: 'In January 1994, the BMA Council approved in principle the concept of limited legislation to translate the common law into statute and clarify the non-liability of doctors who act in accordance with an advance directive'.
36. The Law Commission, Consultation Paper No. 129, *Mentally incapacitated adults and decision-making: medical treatment and research*, para. 3.8. HMSO, London (1993).
37. *Re C* High Court of Justice, Family Division, 14 October 1993 (transcript). In this case the court held that the decision of a schizophrenic to refuse life-saving treatment then, and at any time in the future, was valid.
38. Per Mr Justice Thorpe, p. 9.
39. Adopted at the Plenary Assembly, Cascais, 12–13 November 1993. CP93/83, recommendation 4.
40. Note 35, p. 1.

41. Note 14, p. 54, para 264.
42. Note 14, p. 54, para 265.
43. I am grateful to Chris Docker of the Voluntary Euthanasia Society of Scotland for bringing this to my attention.
44. Note 8, p. 8.
45. Stevens, C. and Hassan, R. (1994). Management of death, dying and euthanasia: attitudes and practices of medical practitioners in South Australia, *Journal of Medical Ethics*, 20, 41.
46. Note 45, p. 45.
47. Mayo, T. (1990). Constitutionalizing the 'right to die'. *Maryland Law Review*, 49, 103.
48. Note 47, p. 144.
49. Lynn, J. and Teno, J. (1993). After the patient self-determination act: the need for empirical research on formal advance directives. *Hastings Center Report*, 23, 20.
50. Note 49, p. 23.
51. Wolf, S.M. (1990). Nancy Beth Cruzan: in no voice at all. *Hastings Center Report*, 20, 41.

6

Outcome Scoring in Intensive Care

Sydney Jacobs

1. Introduction

The care of the critically ill has become increasingly complex and expensive.[1,2] We are able to keep patients with a hopeless prognosis alive for many weeks by artificial support. One retrospective analysis demonstrated that about 20 per cent of patients admitted to an intensive care unit (ICU) had no chance of ultimate survival.[3] Due to the enormous expenses incurred in the ICU we must be careful how we allot this scarce resource. We have duties not only to present but also to future patients,[4,5] and new methods of assessment to meet this challenge are required.

Ideally, in order to define any patient's chance of success on referral we require a pre-admission assessment of outcome. However, this assessment is lacking in respect to most patients referred to a general ICU because this is difficult to make. The reason for this relates to the factors (Table 6.1) that determine outcome.[6] A specific diagnosis is often lacking on referral of patients and certainly the response to therapy may be impossible to predict. A recent admission to ICU exemplifies this dilemma well. A young man of 27 years with acute myeloid leukaemia was referred with severe dyspnoea and a history of a bone marrow transplant (BMT) and total body irradiation (TBI) six weeks prior to admission. Severe shortness of breath and respiratory failure had developed rapidly 24 hours prior to admission. The chest X-ray showed bilateral exudates consistent with a diagnosis of the adult respiratory distress syndrome (ARDS). The patient was commenced on artificial ventilation and antibiotics to cover for atypical bacterial, fungal, and viral organisms. High-dose steroids were also commenced as the consultant haematologist considered the illness might be an example of graft-versus-host disease. The patient also suffered from hepatic and renal dysfunction. The patient made an unexpectedly rapid recovery and was discharged in a satisfactory state from ICU within 72 hours of admission. The cause of the acute illness in this case was unknown and the response to treatment was totally unexpected. The patient on referral was assumed to have ARDS. In retrospect, he clearly did not have ARDS, but what was the cause of his pulmonary oedema? Echocardiography excluded a cardiac cause for the oedema and he was not obviously fluid-overloaded. Some

Table 6.1 Determinants of outcome in critical illness (modified from Knaus *et al.* (1988)[6]

Information availability	Patient and treatment factors
Pre-admission	• Type of disease
	• Severity of disease
	• Physiological reserve
Post-admission	• Response to therapy
	• Type of therapy available
	• Timing and quality of care
	• Adverse events to therapeutic interventions

ICUs might have denied this patient admission knowing the awful prognosis of patients with a combination of ARDS, haematological malignancy, and bone marrow transplant. If he had been denied admission he would certainly have died.

Due to the obvious difficulties in deciding on the suitability of admission of patients referred for intensive care only very broad basic guidelines can be given in formulating an ICU admission policy. This will include patients who require support of their vital systems, in most cases involving the artificial support of ventilation, which cannot be provided on the general wards. However, the policy will exclude terminally ill patients for whom continued provision of the best medical care would offer no reasonable prospect of meaningful recovery. Patients with terminal malignancy and those who are severely compromised neurologically also fit into this latter category. It has been suggested[7] that every patient on admission to hospital should be classified by the patient's responsible consultant or his deputy into three categories:

(1) full support including cardiopulmonary resuscitation (CPR);

(2) full support excluding CPR;

(3) modified support excluding CPR.

If a patient is placed in categories (2) or (3) the situation must be discussed with the patient's relatives. Apart from those groups of patients where the future quality of life is very poor most doctors responsible for admissions take the view that if a referred patient has a chance of survival then that patient should be admitted. In order to provide all patients who can benefit from ICU with the highest standard of care we must be rapidly able to define those patients who can no longer benefit. Withdrawal of treatment from critically ill patients who have no chance of survival is important both from an economic and humanitarian perspective. Nurses and patients' relatives become demoralized by the artificial support of patients who have no hope for ultimate survival. The problem is in deciding in the case of any individual patient that their condition has become hopeless. There is generally a reluctance by doctors to withdraw support from those patients whose prognosis has become hopeless. This reluctance has been blamed on doctors' uncertainty, acute awareness of their fallibility,[8] and possible medico-legal implications. The cost involved in maintaining treatment of patients with a hopeless prognosis is enormous—'If unnecessary care was largely eliminated, not only would the cost of medical care be reduced but the rate of increase of that cost would be reduced'.[9]

As pre-admission indices of outcome are lacking in the majority of patients, scoring systems have been devised that can define the severity of illness either on admission or after 24 hours of admission.[10–15] Outcome predictions, for so long neglected in medical practice,[16] have now become recognized as an important component of medical management. The omission of prediction from the major goals of basic medical science has compromised the intellectual content of clinical work since a modern clinician's main challenge in the care of patients is to make predictions.[16] However, many clinicians remain unaware of, or sceptical about, the potential value of objective prediction or probability estimates in clinical practice. This scepticism derives partly from a feeling of unease at the possibility of being influenced by a computer's prediction, but more cogently from the clinician's knowledge of important features of a patient's illness that are not incorporated in the prediction model, and from awareness that the ability to predict death with absolute accuracy is an impossibility.

The use of scoring systems to predict outcome in critically ill patients is very recent. Severity of illness is the single most important factor that predicts outcome of patients receiving ICU treatment.[17] Scoring systems are essential if stratification of patients into severity of illness is required for audit and resource management, to compare institutions, to study different methods of treatment in clinical trials and eventually to predict individual outcomes. With all scoring systems meticulous data collection is required and should be carried out by trained observers. Scoring systems can be defined into two broad categories: static and dynamic. Static scoring systems can be further divided into numerical and multivariate models which in turn may have specific or general application.

2. Static scoring systems

Numerical scores applicable to all patient groups

The numerical scores rely on the judgment of experts to identify the principal indicators involved in the index, to weight and suggest measures. Gustafson has discussed the significance of multi-attribute utility theory in relation to a valid judgemental approach to index development and has discussed and made recommendations for the development of scoring systems.[18] Sets of factors which are considered important for judging the severity of illness are identified. Experts suggest measures of assessing each factor and subjectively estimate weights for each factor. Each factor is converted into a common utility measurement scale that reflects the relative contribution of each to the total severity assessment of the patient. The severity score for a patient with a specific combination of those factors is calculated by summing the weighted components. This approach does not rely on outcome data for construction of the index. The effect of severity is separated from the effect of treatment. Such judgemental methods are quick and relatively inexpensive and as good as mathematically derived diagnostic models produced from an empiric database.[18] Judgementally derived indexes are easily modified and repeatable. Expert physicians are better able to control for quality when making severity assessments.

Therapeutic Intervention Score. This scoring system[10,11] monitors the amount of therapy needed to support the patient. It was the first scoring system to be applicable to the broad case mix of ICU patients. The rationale for its creation was the great concern at the vast expenditure generated in the ICU area. The system classifies the severity of illness by quantifying the degree of therapeutic intervention. The more ill the patient the more therapy is required. Therapeutic interventions are scored on a 1 to 4 range according to the time and effort required for nursing care. The system represents an initial stage in the development of stratification of critical illness but it cannot be used as a predictive instrument as the use of therapy will vary greatly from one institution to another and within institutions over time. It has been useful in investigating costs in the ICU.[19]

Acute and Chronic Health Evaluation (APACHE). The APACHE II severity of disease system described by Knaus and his colleagues[13] is by far the most widespread scoring system in use. An understanding of how the scoring system is derived, the meaning of its various components, and limitations is crucial for its application. Knaus *et al.*[12] suggested that the severity of illness could be assessed by measuring the degree of abnormality of several physiological variables. They initially defined an Acute Physiological Score (APS) derived from points appropriate for the degree of abnormality of 34 variables. The aim of this system was to attempt to predict hospital mortality in patient groups and later to consider refinement to predict individual outcome. Selection and weighting of physiological variables depended on expert opinion. Such a system is objective and independent of treatment. The weighted system is based on a 0 to 4 scale. The APS is derived from the worst (most deranged) physiological value during the first 24 hours of ICU admission. Use of the 24-hour period ensures that all values are available. Clinical judgement is

Table 6.2 APACHE II system (after Knaus *et al.* 1985)[13]

Parameter	Value range	Score	Parameter	Value range	Score
Core temperature	0 –29.9	4	Plasma potassium	0 –2.4	4
(°C)	30.0–31.9	3	(mmol/l)	2.5–2.9	2
	32.0–33.9	2		3.0–3.4	1
	34.0–35.9	1		3.5–5.4	0
	36.0–38.9	0		5.5–5.9	1
	38.5–38.9	1		6.0–6.9	3
	39.0–40.9	3		7.0 or more	4
	41 or more	4		7.0 or more	4
Heart rate	0– 39	4	Plasma creatinine	0– 52	2
(per min)	40– 54	3	(μmol/l)	53–132	0
	55– 69	2	Double points for	133–176	2
	70–109	0	acute renal failure	177–308	3
	110–139	2		309 or more	4
	140–179	3			
	180 or more	4			
Mean blood	0– 49	4	Arterial pH	0 –7.14	4
pressure	50– 69	2		7.15–7.24	3
(mmHg)*	70–109	0		7.25–7.32	2
	110–129	2		7.33–7.49	0
	130–159	3		7.50–7.59	1
	160 or more	4	or:	7.60–7.69	3
			(if no blood gases)	7.7 or more	4
Respiratory rate	0– 5	4	Venous bicarbonate	0 –14.9	4
(per min)	6– 9	2	(mmol/l)	15.0–17.9	3
	10–11	1		18.0–21.9	2
(Omit if	12–24	0		22.0–31.9	0
ventilated)	25–34	1		32.0–40.9	1
	35–49	3		41.0–51.9	3
	50 or more	4		52 or more	4
White cell count	0 – 0.9	4	Arterial Po_2	0 –7.32	4
(multi 10°/l)	1.0– 2.9	2	kPa	7.33–8.12	3
	3.0–14.9	0	(inspired O_2<50%)	8.13–9.33	1
	15.0–19.9	1	or:	9.34 & over	0
	20.0–39.9	2			
	0.0 or more	4			

Table 6.2 continued

Parameter	Value range	Score	Parameter	Value range	Score
Haematocrit	0 –19.9	4	Alveolar/Arterial	0 –26.6	0
(%)	20.0–29.9	2	P_{O_2} DIFFERENCE	26.7–46.6	2
	30.0–45.9	0	kPa (P_A–P_a>O_2)	46.7–66.6	3
	46.0–49.9	1	(inspired O_2>50 %)	66.7 & over	4
	50.0–59.9	2	Age	0–44	0
	60 or more	4	(years)	45–54	2
				55–64	3
				65–74	5
				75 or more	6
Plasma sodium	0–110	4	GLASGOW COMA SCORE (15–actual score)		
(mmol/l)	111–119	3	Organ failure/immunosuppression		
	120–129	2	*Cardiac*: New York Heart Ass. Grade IV		
	130–149	0	*Respiratory*: minimal effort dyspnoea		
	150–154	1	*Hepatic cirrhosis/portal hypertension*		
	155–159	2	*Renal*: receiving chronic dialysis.		
	160–179	3	Any immunodeficiency/suppression.		
	180 or more	4	(Post-elective surgery, score 2; for		
			acute surgery/non-operative, score 5)		

˙Mean arterial blood pressure = (2 × diastolic) plus (systolic)/3.

required to ensure all values are correct. The APS is combined with weighting for age and chronic ill health reflecting the physiological reserve of the patient. The combination of APS, age, and chronic ill health, gives the APACHE score. The higher the score the greater the severity of illness and the greater the risk of hospital death.

The complexity of the original scoring system using 34 variables suggested that simplification was required. Subsequently a simplified version known as APACHE II was developed.[13] This new version was produced by excluding any variable on clinical judgement and evaluating it using multivariate comparison. By this means it was found that the smallest number of variables that reflected physiological derangement for all vital organs whilst maintaining statistical precision was 12 (Table 6.2). The importance of renal function for outcome determined that the threshold at which creatinine contributed to a score was changed and weighting doubled for acute renal failure. The scoring range for each variable is shown in Table 6.2. The maximum APACHE II score attainable is 71.

The APACHE II severity of disease classification system was validated in 13 American hospitals among nearly 6000 patients. The most specific standard for judging the validity of severity scoring is hospital mortality as this can be

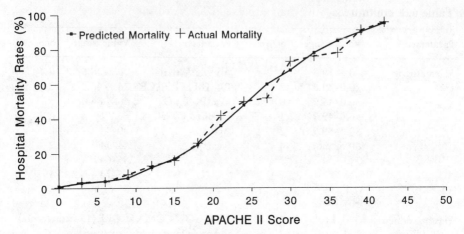

Fig. 6.1 Mortality rate and APPACHE II scoring. Data from 5030 consecutive patients admitted to the ICU at 13 hospitals. Actual (– – – –) and predicted (————) mortality rates are indicated (gamma = 0.995) (after Knaus *et al.* 1986).[20]

accurately and simply measured but it has the disadvantage that it gives no indication of the important factor of quality of life. It was shown that for each 5-point increase in APACHE II score there was a significant increase in hospital death rate (Fig. 6.1). It was also evident that the overall risk of hospital death rate varied according to the disease. For example, patients with congestive cardiac failure admitted with APACHE II scores 10 to 19 had a hospital death rate half that of patients with septic shock in the same score band. As the risk of death varies with the disease process as well as the severity of illness the APACHE II risk of death was devised.[13] The risk of death is a probability of hospital death expressed as a percentage. This can be derived from a multiple logistic regression equation appropriate for the analysis of a dichotomous outcome, such as mortality prediction. It can be calculated from a knowledge of the APACHE II score, specific disease process, or major system involvement, and the necessity of emergency surgery. The risk of death is calculated from the following formula:

Natural log (*R*/1 minus *R*) = minus 3.517 plus (APACHE II score multiplied by 0.146) plus 0.0603 (only if post-emergency surgery) plus diagnostic category weights where *R* = Risk of hospital death.

For groups of critically ill patients the predicted or expected death rate is computed by summing all the Risks of Death from the equation above and dividing by the number of patients. The mortality ratio (MR) of a group of patients can be obtained by dividing the actual by the expected mortality. An MR <1 indicates that fewer deaths have occurred, whereas an MR >1 tells us that there are more deaths than expected relative to the reference data set; it tells us nothing more than that. It tells us nothing, for example, about the quality of the ICU. A knowledge of the organization and clinical processes of the ICU, as well as subgroup analyses, are required before inferences can be made. Even then any inference is only a hypothesis that requires further testing. Knaus used the MR to compare the performance of thirteen American hospitals.[20]

Knaus also investigated the prognosis in patients with multiple organ failure.[21] Organ failure criteria were obtained by a review of the literature and modified by expert agreement. Prognosis in organ system failure is related to the number and duration of organ system failures (OSF) as shown in Table 6.3.

Knaus considered that cardiac surgical patients, including those for coronary artery bypass, were in many ways unique.[13] This is perhaps due to physiological abnormalities present after bypass spontaneously reverting to normal, masking by multiple system support devices, and by occurrence of unexpected events post-operatively. APACHE II was anticipated to be a poor predictor of outcome in these patients and cardiac surgical patients were not included in Knaus's original patient cohort. For ICUs with a high throughput of post-operative coronary artery bypass surgery it was advised that these patients should be excluded when comparisons are being made with ICUs without such patients. This system was subsequently evaluated[22] among a large number of patients undergoing cardiothoracic surgery and, in fact, has demonstrated a good relationship between the score and mortality rate. APACHE II scores have also been correlated with mortality in 100 patients hospitalized for general peritonitis or abdominal abscess.[23] This study prospectively validated pre-treatment APACHE II scoring in abdominal sepsis.

Although this scoring system has been shown to be simple and robust there have been practical problems associated with its use. All the variables, with the exception of the neurological score, are objective. There are difficulties associated with the neurological score which are compounded by it being heavily weighted. Patients are frequently intubated, sedated, and perhaps paralysed and occasionally deaf, making interpretation of the Glasgow Coma Scale (GCS) difficult or impossible. Some workers[24] use the best GCS and others overestimate neurological deficit by accepting the worst value over the 24-hour period, failing to allow for the effect of drugs, etc., so that their patients have a high score but a good outcome.

Tertiary referral hospitals may be compromised in regard to outcome of their patients if they take a large number of referrals from other ICUs compared to others which do not.[25] This suggests that it is important to record the exact timing of the onset of ICU treatment. Selection bias as well as lead time bias must also be considered when analysing the results of group data.[26]

The APACHE II Risk of Death also presents a dilemma because it relies on a subjective choice on admission of a specific diagnostic category or major organ

Table 6.3 Mortality related to the number and duration of major organ system failures (OSFs) (after Knaus et al. 1985)[21]

No.			Day of failure						
			1st	2nd	3rd	4th	5th	6th	7th
1	Per cent mortality		22%	31%	34%	35%	40%	42%	41%
	No. deaths	450		261	204	159	142	118	80
	No. patients	2070		847	607	455	356	279	195
2	Per cent mortality		52%	67%	66%	62%	56%	64%	68%
	No. deaths	239		147	103	118	96	78	56
	No. patients	458		219	156	191	171	122	82
3	Per cent mortality		80%	95%	93%	96%	100%	100%	100%
	No. deaths	152		70	50	50	38	33	32
	No. patients	191		74	54	52	38	33	32

system involvement. The coefficients to be chosen assume a knowledge of the exact problem of a patient on admission. This knowledge is frequently absent in the case of patients seen in a general ICU. Weighting for a prediction of outcome is wholly dependent on the diagnosis or major organ system involvement being known. Even if the diagnosis is known the diagnostic categories are not easy to use in many cases and they are not comprehensive. Expected outcome calculations as one would expect from this situation are subject to inter-observer variation. One report[27] showed that it was the exception for two doctors to agree on the estimated risk of hospital death and in one patient the risk ranged from 18 to 56 per cent. Scoring has been used in specific patient groups and compared with specific scoring systems. In some cases, for example, in the assessment and monitoring of acute pancreatitis, APACHE II performed better than Ranson[28] and Imrie[29] scoring in predicting outcome.[30] Similarly, in the adult respiratory distress syndrome, APACHE II with correction for number and duration of organ system failure[31] outperformed the ventilatory index.[32] Combinations of scoring systems may complement the APACHE II scoring,[33] as demonstrated with the Trauma[34] and Injury Severity Scores.[35] On the other hand, the Critical Care Scoring system incorporating haemodynamic, oxygen transport, and perfusion measurements was found to predict outcome more accurately than APACHE II, although patients studied were presented for invasive monitoring.[36]

APACHE II can measure severity of illness accurately. One of the best goodness of fit tests is to determine the area under the receiver-operator characteristic (ROC) curve.[13] The ROC curve shows the relationship between sensitivity and specificity at different cut-off points. A perfect scoring system will produce a right-angled line whereas one which is unable to differentiate between the two populations will produce a diagonal line. The area under the right angle in the case of the APACHE II score is in excess of 85 percent. The APACHE II system can also be used to estimate risk in groups of patients for the purposes of audit and clinical trials, provided the groups are large enough (i.e. more than 100). The MR should always be quoted together with the 95 per cent confidence interval.

The score has now been refined using data collected from 17 440 ICU admissions in 40 units to produce APACHE III.[37] There are now five new variables included (urine output, serum albumin, urea, bilirubin, and glucose). Pre-ICU admission location is defined. Serum potassium and bicarbonate are dispensed with. There is modification of the neurological score and acid base components. Increased accuracy results from the expansion of 0 to 4 weights to larger score variations, and redefinement of acid base assessment. The maximum score is now 299. More diagnostic categories are incorporated for the calculation of the mortality risk and are said to give estimates within 3 per cent of that observed in 95 per cent of patients. It will take some time for this new version to be independently assessed.

Simplified Acute Physiological Score (SAPS).   This score[14] was developed in France. It is very similar to Acute Physiological Score of APACHE II but excludes chronic ill health and diagnostic data. It is simpler and less time-consuming than APACHE II but cannot easily be converted to a probability of hospital mortality.

Numerical scores applicable to specific patient groups

Glasgow Coma Scale (GCS).   This scale[38] examines the impact of injury or disease on the central nervous system. It was one of the earlier scoring systems to achieve international recognition. It measures the depth of coma following head injury and when used over time it can give an indication of improvement or deterioration in the acute phase as well as predicting ultimate outcome. The following aspects of behaviour are independently measured: motor response, verbal performance, and eye opening. There was an evident need for such a system because previous systems for describing patients with impaired consciousness were inconsistent and this naturally caused confusion when patients were exchanged between hospitals and clinical trials were carried out. Responses are identified that can be clearly defined and accurately graded according to a rank order that indicates the degree of dysfunction. In practice it has high consistency and ambiguities are small. Assessing the severity of head injuries is difficult and requires attention to the following features: initial status, neurological complications, duration of coma, post-traumatic amnesia, and, finally, physical and mental sequelae. Sequelae can be assessed according to the Glasgow Outcome Scale (GOS)[39] which enables surviving patients to be classified according to social outcome. Prognostic information has been derived from a data bank of more than 1000 patients with head injuries by relating the severity of the initial insult to subsequent outcome.[40] Levy *et al.*[41] have applied similar techniques to predict outcome from non traumatic coma and to suggest individual prognosis after cardiac arrest.[42]

Injury Severity and Trauma Scores.   Well-known and utilized measures of the severity of trauma are the Injury Severity (ISS) and Trauma Scores (TS) which retrospectively grade trauma at various sites of the body[35] or by physiological severity.[34] An Abbreviated Injury Scale (AIS)[43,44] was initially used. Injuries are assigned a six-digit code based on their anatomical site and severity. The sixth digit represents the AIS severity score, rating injury by increasing severity from 1–6. The first five digits identify the specific injury. The ISS equals the sum of the squares of the AIS from the three most severely injured body regions. Scoring is carried out in six possible areas which include the head and neck, face, abdominal and pelvic contents, chest, bony pelvis and limbs, and body surface. Use of ISS shows good correlation with mortality and shows the effect of injuries that would not themselves be life-threatening unless accompanied by other injuries.[45] It should be noted that the ISS in non-linear and non-parametric statistics should be used for analysis.

The TS was developed from the Triage Index[46] as a measure of injury severity and based on five variables. Further developments have produced a modified version of the TS known as the Revised Trauma Score (RTS)[47] which uses a weighted sum of the coded values of only three variables: systolic blood pressure, respiratory rate, and GCS. A further refinement to improve prediction of outcome was achieved by combination of the RTS with ISS, age, and type of injury to produce the TRISS method.[48] Yet another refinement known as a Severity Characterization of Trauma combines admission values of RTS variables, age of patient, type of injury, and a new characterization of the anatomical lesions.[49] These various scores have been tested and compared for their predictive performance in patient groups.[50,51] APACHE II, ISS, and TS performed similarly in patients but accuracy increased when they were combined.[52]

Burn Index. This index[53] incorporates the total area burned and the age of the patient. This is an example of a simple and good pre-treatment index of risk of death. However, these two indices of burn mortality can never fully describe this complex problem. We require at least another four indices to describe the situation.[54] These include Pa_{O2}, presence or absence of airway oedema, percentage of third degree burn, and the presence of prior bronchopulmonary disease.

Ventilatory Index (VI). This index was developed by Smith and Gordon[32] as a possible predictor of outcome in patients with the adult respiratory distress syndrome (ARDS) and to be a practical guide for triage in the ICU. These authors suggested that two physiological variables: the alveolar arterial oxygen gradient (AaD_{O2}) and the peak airway pressure, together with age were predictive of outcome. However, none of their patients with a VI over 80 survived. ARDS is often the result of a severe systemic catastrophe, such as septic shock, and thus may be better assessed by a general scoring system which incorporates all organ systems.[31]

Multivariate statistical models applicable to all patient groups

The multivariate statistical approach develops indices intended to correlate with an outcome statistic. However, outcome is a function of both severity and quality of care. The quality of care will determine the correlation between outcome and severity. Outcome-based severity indices may confuse quality and severity. The system relies on a database which is difficult and expensive to collect. Databases, even large ones, are sensitive to the particular database being used and may be suspect in other populations. The advantages are that this approach reduces a large number of potential outcome predictors to a small subset and the assigned weights of the selected variables are determined objectively.

Mortality prediction model (MPM).   This model (MPM) is an objective method described by Lemeshow *et al.*[55] and Teres *et al.*[56] using multiple logistic regression methods to estimate probability of mortality. The chosen variables and the weighting of each were determined by computerized statistical procedures applied to a database of 755 consecutive ICU patients. This data base was used to predict hospital mortality at the time of admission and after 24 hours. Two models were initially described. One considered the use of cardiopulmonary resuscitation prior to admission and the other the number of organ failures on admission. Both were based on seven variables. Predicted outcome with the two models on admission were closely correlated with actual outcome. The 24-hour model, however, could not be validated. The most recent version of the system[57] employs 11 binary variables (requiring yes/no responses); these include emergency or previous ICU admission, age, coma, previous cardio-pulmonary arrest, chronic renal failure, cancer, infection, systolic blood pressure, heart rate, and surgery. It shows excellent goodness-of-fit, sensitivity, specificity, and correct classification rate. It has been tested against APACHE II and SAPS and most closely matched the observed outcome compared with the other systems.[58]

Although the MPM has been validated in a study population independent of that in which it was developed it has not undergone the very widespread international validation of APACHE II. Its advantages are that it is treatment-independent, provides useful prognostic data and can stratify patient groups at the time of admission.

Multivariate models applicable to specific patient groups

Multivariate techniques have been used previously for patients with circulatory failure[59] and drug overdose,[60] and have been proposed for patients with chest pain[61] for triage to a coronary care unit.

Cardiovascular system.   Work by Shoemaker[62] has shown that multivariate nonparametric statistical analysis provides methods to predict outcome early in hypovolaemic shock in the post-operative period and most importantly to define therapeutic goals. A predictive index based on probability distribution of various variables gives an overall predictive index which serves as a quantitative measure of the severity of illness expressed in statistical terms that reflect the likelihood of survival. Good outcome prognostic capability was determined for left ventricular stroke work index, oxygen delivery, and oxygen consumption.

Chronic hepatic failure.   Work by Garden[63] showed that three variables: the initial prothrombin time ratio, serum creatinine, and the presence or absence of encephalopathy, were independently predictive of outcome and using them in a derived regression equation they were able to demonstrate that a probability of discharge figure of 0.66 divided the high-risk patient from the low-risk patient. They successfully predicted outcome in 90 per cent of their admissions. Subsequent work has suggested that the prothrombin time ratio alone may be more predictive of outcome.[64]

3. Dynamic scoring systems

No static scoring systems can help us with a clinical decision to withdraw therapy for individual ICU patients as they do not provide sufficient information to define the features distinguishing survivors from non-survivors. Chang *et al.*,[65] Jacobs *et al.*,[66] and Bion *et al.*[67] were the first to explore the possibility of utilizing a dynamic scoring system for outcome prediction in individual patients. Initially, two APACHE II scores over time were used for this purpose to help identify those patients who would not benefit from total parenteral nutrition (TPN).[65] Sensitivity (defined as predicted dead, dead/predicted dead, dead plus unknown prediction, dead) greatly improved with two scores. Bion *et al.*[68] using the sickness score, a modified APACHE II score, also showed that a day 4 score improved the predictive power, and failure to obtain a reduction in score was associated with an increased risk of death. Subsequently, daily APACHE II scores were used to define patterns of change which were associated with non-survival.[8]

There are theoretical and practical reasons why a day 1 APACHE II assessment is inadequate for making outcome predictions:[8]

1. The pathophysiological processes affecting ICU patients are dynamic and cannot be reflected by a single assessment on the day of admission to the ICU.

2. Although the APACHE II score, with the exception of the neurological score, is based on objective data, derivation of the risk of death depends on a subjective choice of a single specific diagnostic category or major organ system as the primary cause of admission. The exact choice can frequently be difficult to make, not only on the day of admission but also subsequently. This problem is especially true of patients in multi-organ failure. An incorrect choice can lead to a wrong estimation of death and therefore a wrong prediction.

3. The APACHE II Risk of Death is a probability obtained by applying coefficients to the APACHE II score. The coefficients are derived data obtained from the first day of admission. The risk of death may therefore not be valid for analysis over time.

4. Patients commonly develop other major organ system failures during their stay in the ICU with important prognostic implications.

5. Major clinical decisions would never be acceptable to clinicians, patients, and their relatives if based only on a single assessment.

In order to develop a dynamic model to identify individual patients who will die during the course of their illness some important considerations must be mentioned.[69] Strategically, it is important to make a prediction of death and not survival. A patient admitted to the ICU will have an unknown outcome. The aim of treatment is to achieve survival and this continues as long as outcome remains unknown. When death is considered to have become inevitable all treatment is stopped and the consequences of that decision become irreversible.

There are three questions to be answered when considering the features which distinguish survivors from non-survivors:[69]

1. What is the cause of death of most ICU patients?

2. Are there markers of this process?

3. Are there reproducible patterns of these markers?

Most ICU patients die from multiple organ failure. Daily organ failure scoring (OFS) which is daily APACHE II scoring with correction for the number and the duration of organ failures, can be used to define the pathophysiological status and its daily rate of change.[8] Organ failure coefficients used in calculating the OFS from the number and duration of organ failures were values obtained by dividing the mortality rates quoted by Knaus,[21] shown in Table 6.3, by 1000. The rate of change of the physiological status is important information in identifying the progress of any patient. To follow these changes in pathophysiological status a computer system has been developed.[8,69] It allows dynamic analysis of the change in OFS. The program analyses the rate of change of OFS compared to that of the previous day and the absolute value of the OFS over the window of two days. Two patterns of change (Figs 6.2 & 6.3) were recognized in non-survivors but not in survivors. The original training set comprised 310 consecutive ICU patients whose outcomes were followed until death or discharge from hospital. Daily OFS improved the predictive power compared to a single or daily APACHE II score by a factor of 5.3 and 1.4, respectively. Once a prediction of death is made on a patient that prediction holds even if the score decreases. The Riyadh predictive algorithm (Fig. 6.4) was further tested prospectively on a larger cohort of 830 consecutive ICU patients. It correctly predicted 38 per cent (109/290) of non-survivors and there were no false predictions of death. The importance of these predictions can be seen by their timing and effect on bed usage (Table 6.4). In the UK the mean daily cost in an ICU varies between £550 for survivors to £816 for non-survivors (95 per cent confidence interval £498–606 and £609–982 respectively).[70] Therefore, the potential saving by withdrawing treatment on the day the computer predicted non-survival would have been substantial. It is important to appreciate, however, that these predictions were never used clinically to withdraw treatment from any patient. Data was taken prospectively but analysed retrospectively after the patients had died or

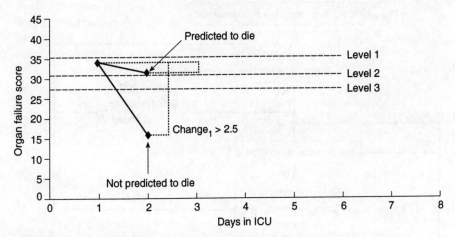

Fig. 6.2 Dynamic analysis of organ failure scores for days 1 or 2 in the ICU. If a patient scores 31–35 points on day 1, and the score does not improve by more than 2.5 points, the patient is predicted to die (after Chang *et al.* 1988).[8]

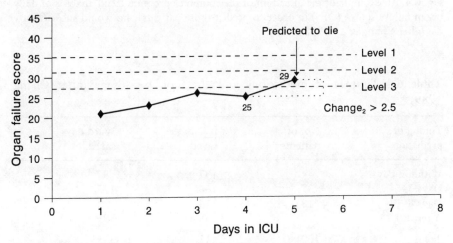

Fig. 6.3 Dynamic analysis of organ failure score for day 2 and onwards in the ICU. If a patient's score increases by more than 2.5 points, and the absolute value is greater than 27 points, the patient is predicted to die (after Chang *et al.* 1988).[8]

been discharged from hospital. The predictions by the Riyadh algorithm were shown in one clinical study to be superior to those based on clinical experience and judgment.[71] The assessment of individual patient predictions can best be performed by the False Positive Diagnosis Rate (FPDR = false predictions of death/total predictions of death). In this study, the ability of

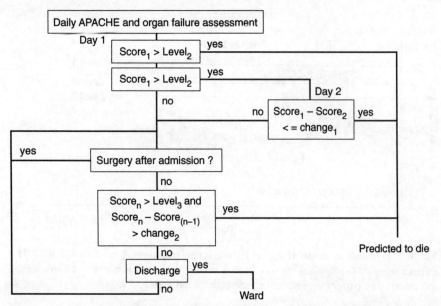

Fig. 6.4 An example of the alorithm of the computer program trend analysis of daily organ failure scores (OFS) in order to predict those patients who would subsequently die (after Chang *et al.* 1988).[8]

Table 6.4 Timings of predictions and effect on bed usage (after Chang 1989)[69]

Timing of prediction	No. of patients	ICU days saved	Ward days saved
Within 2 days	44	197	87
Days 3–7	37	166	125
Days 8–14	18	114	24
After day 14	10	38	99
Total	109	515	335

Days saved = time between prediction of death and subsequent death, with the assumption that if treatment had been withdrawn, death would have occurred within 24 hours.

doctors and nurses to make early predictions of death showed that the FPDR of clinicians varied between 9 per cent and 16 per cent compared to zero per cent for the computer's predictions.

The Riyadh predictive algorithm has been shown in one institution to identify 38 per cent of non-survivors although a more recent study[72] has shown that this figure may not be representative of ICUs in general. This study carried out in a UK teaching hospital demonstrated that only 16 per cent (34/209) of the hospital non-survivors were predicted to die by the computer but of more concern in this group were three patients falsely predicted to die. In the Cardiff study, the FPDR and specificity (unknown predictions surviving/total survivors) were 8.8 per cent and 99.6 per cent respectively. This demonstrates that the FPDR and not the specificity best reflects the performance of a score for individual outcome predictions.

In practice, can we use the Riyadh predictive algorithm with the help of a computer to avoid useless intensive care? Are the predictions accurate enough? The accuracy of the Riyadh data is certainly impressive (i.e. no false predictions and a sensitivity of about 38 per cent). The Cardiff data using the Riyadh algorithm, were less impressive with a FPDR of death of 8.8 per cent and a sensitivity of only 15 per cent. The false-positive prediction of death when experienced doctors and nurses were compared with the Riyadh algorithm varied between 9 per cent and 16 per cent. The Second European Consensus Conference[73] considered existing scores unsuitable for individual patient predictions but observed that dynamic scores which identify trends in illness severity can improve the accuracy of existing models. With dynamic scoring individual predictions have become more feasible.

Some physicians have suggested that greater efforts should be expended in trying to derive better treatment rather than predictive algorithms. The answer to this argument is that both approaches are relevant and important. Future refinements to improve prediction may include pattern recognition algorithms with increased time windows. Some combinations of organ failures do worse than others. This could be taken into account by appropriate coefficients. Chronic health points are crude and do not allow for gradations in severity of disease.

The APACHE III daily risk assessment[37] which gives a probability of death is derived from data collected over seven days and thereafter the equation is 're-cycled'. In comparison, the Riyadh individual outcome prediction algorithm data is collected until discharge or death. APACHE III is based on regression equations and thus does not have the ability to track the trends of individual patients. The other problem with this system for obtaining daily risk assessments is the same as that with the day 1 risk of death already noted. An exact diagnosis is required to obtain the appropriate coefficient and thus to calculate correctly the risk of death. Many ICU patients defy diagnostic categorization. There are no studies yet reported where individual outcome probabilities using APACHE III have been tested on a prospective set of patients.

7. Conclusion

At present, there is no system that has been devised to triage admissions into the intensive care unit for treatment. Specific admission policies for the ICU are inappropriate and require only very general guidelines. Once a patient is admitted it is important for humanitarian and economic reasons to recognize rapidly hopelessly ill patients so that they can be allowed to die with dignity and with freedom from pain as they approach the end of their lives. The introduction of economic considerations for individual patient outcome decisions is a difficult dilemma but one which will become increasingly necessary to confront as society is forced to debate on the most effective use of its limited health resources. Computerized predictions of outcome from trends of daily severity scoring may support a clinical decision in the future but this process must be under the control of experienced medical personnel who fully understand its function, its dangers, and the many pitfalls.

Notes

1. Riffin, T.A. (1989). Intensive care unit survival of patients with systemic illness. *American Reviews of Respiratory Diseases*, 1, 328–35.
2. Shiell, A., Griffiths, R.D., Macmillan, R.R., and Atherton, S.T. (1989). Pilot assessment of the cost effectiveness of a British intensive therapy unit. *British Journal of Health Medicine*, 42, 144–5.
3. Jacobs, S., Chang, R.W.S., Lee, B., and Lee, B. (1989). An analysis of the utilisation of an intensive care unit. *Intensive Care Medicine*, 15, 511–18.
4. Hiatt, H.M. (1975). Protecting the medical commons: who is responsible? *New England Journal of Medicine*, 293, 235–41.
5. Jecker, N.S. and Pearlman, R.A. (1992). Medical futility who decides? *Archives of Internal Medicine*, 152, 1140–4.
6. Knaus, W.A., *et al.* (1988). The science of prediction and its implications for the clinician to-day. *Theoretical Surgery*, 3, 93–101.
7. Davila, F., Boisaubin, E.U., and Sears, D.A. (1986). Patient care categories: an approach to do-not-resuscitate decisions in a public teaching hospital. *Critical Care Medicine*, 14, 1066–7.
8. Chang, R.W.S., Jacobs, S., and Lee, B. (1988). Predicting outcome among intensive care unit patients using computerised trend analysis of daily Apache II scores corrected for organ system failure. *Intensive Care Medicine*, 14, 558–66.
9. Angell, M. (1985). Cost containment and the physician. *Journal of the American Medical Association*, 254, 1203–7.
10. Cullen, D.J., *et al.* (1974). Therapeutic intervention scoring system: A method for quantitative comparison of patient care. *Critical Care Medicine*, 2, 57–62.
11. Keene, R.A. and Cullen D.J. (1983). Therapeutic intervention scoring system: Update 1983. *Critical Care Medicine*, 11, 1–3.
12. Knaus, W.A., *et al.* (1981). APACHE—Acute physiological and chronic health evaluation: a physiologically based classification system. *Critical Care Medicine*, 9, 591–7.
13. Knaus, W.A., *et al.* (1985). APACHE II. A severity of disease classification. 13, *Critical Care Medicine*, 13, 818–29.
14. Le Gall, J.R., *et al.* (1984). A simplified acute physiological score for ICU patients. *Critical Care Medicine*, 12, 975–7.
15. Lemeshow S, *et al.* (1985). A method for predicting survival and mortality

of ICU patients using objectively derived weights. *Critical Care Medicine*, 13, 519–25.

16. Feinstein A.R. (1983). An additional basic science for clinical medicine. 1. The constraining fundamental paradigms. *Annals of International Medicine*, 99, 393–7.

17. Knaus, W.A., Wagner, D.P., Zimmerman, J.E., and Draper, E.A. (1993). Variation in hospital mortality and length of stay in intensive care. *Annals of International Medicine*, 118, 753–61.

18. Gustafson, D.H., *et al.* (1983). An evaluation of multiple trauma severity indices created by different index development strategies. *Medical Care* 21, 674–91.

19. Slatyer, M.A., James, O.F., Moore, P.G., and Leeder, S.R. (1986). Costs, severity of illness and outcome in intensive care. *Anaethesia in Intensive Care*, 14, 381–9.

20. Knaus, W.A., *et al.* (1986). An evaluation of outcome from intensive care in major medical Centers. 104, 410–8. 104, 410–8.

21. Knaus, W.A., *et al.* (1985). Prognosis in acute organ failure. *Annals of Surgery*, 202, 685–93.

22. Turner, J.S., *et al.* (1991). Acute physiological and chronic health evaluation (APACHE) scoring in a cardiothoracic intensive care unit. *Critical Care Medicine*, 126, 1266–9.

23. Bohnen J.M.A., *et al.* (1988). APACHE II Score and abdominal sepsis: A prospective study. *Archives of Surgery*, 123, 225–9.

24. Jacobs S., Chang R.W.S., Lee B., and Lee B. (1988). Audit of intensive care: a 30 month experience using the APACHE II severity of disease classification. *Intensive Care Medicine*, 14, 567–74.

25. Dragstedt, L., *et al.* (1989). Interhospital comparisons of patient outcome from intensive care: importance of lead-time bias. *Critical Care Medicine*, 17, 418–22.

26. Cerra, F.B., Negro, F., and Abrams, J. (1990). APACHE II score does not predict multiple organ failure or mortality in post-operative surgical patients. *Archives of Surgery*, 125, 519–22.

27. Jackson, E.A., Udwadia, Z.F., Rothwell, P.M., and Lawler, P.G. APACHE II expected outcome calculations are subject to inter-observer variation. (Letter). *Anaesthesia*, 45, 888–9.

28. Ranson, J.H.C., *et al.* (1978). Prognostic signs and the role of operative management in acute pancreatitis. *Surgery, Gynaecology & Obstetrics*, 139, 69–81.

29. Imrie, C.W., *et al.* A single centre double-blind trial of Trasylol therapy in primary acutre pancreatitis. *British Journal of Surgery*, 65, 337–41.

30. Larvin, M. and McMahon M.J. (1989). APACHE II score for assessment and monitoring of acute pancreatitis. *Lancet*, 1, 201–5.

31. Jacobs, S., Chang, R.W.S., and Lee, B. (1991). Prognosis in the adult respiratory distress syndrome: comparison of a ventilatory index with the Riyadh Intensive Care Programme. *Clinics in Intensive Care*, 2, 81–5.

32. Smith, P.E.M. and Gordon, I.J. (1986). An index to predict outcome in adult respiratory distress syndrome. *Intensive Care Medicine*, 43, 923–6.

33. Rhee, K.J., *et al.* (1990). APACHE II scoring in the injured patient. *Critical Care Medicine*, 18, 827–30.

34. Champion H.R., *et al.* (1981). Trauma score. *Critical Care Medicine.*, 9, 672–6.

35. Baker, S.P., O'Neill, B., Haddon, W., and Long, W.B. (1974). The injury severity score: a method for describing patients with multiple injuries and evaluating emergency care. *Journal of Trauma*, 14, 187–96.

36. Yeung, H.C. *et al.* (1990). Critical care scoring system: a concept based on haemodynamic data. *Critical Care Medicine*, 18, 1347–52.

37. Knaus, W.A., *et al.* (1991). The APACHE III prognostic system: risk prediction of hospital mortality for critically ill hospitalised patients. *Chest*, 100, 1619–36.

38. Teasdale, G. and Jennett, B. (1974). Assessment of coma and impaired consciousness. A practical scale. *Lancet*, ii, 81–4.

39. Jennett, B. and Bond, M. (1975). Assessment of outcome after severe brain damage. A practical scale. *Lancet*, i, 480–4.

40. Jennett, B., Teasdale, G., Braakman, R., Minderhoud, J., Heiden, J., and Kurze, T. (1979). Prognosis of patients with severe head injury. *Neurosurgery*, 4, 283–9.

41. Levy, D.E., *et al.* (1981). Prognosis in non-traumatic coma. *Annals of Internal Medicine*, 94, 293–301.

42. Levy, D.E., *et al.* (1985). Predicting outcome from hypoxicischaemic coma. *Journal of the American Medical Association*, 253, 1420–6.

43. Committee on Medical Aspects of Automative Safety. (1971). Rating the severity of tissue damage. 1. The Abbreviated Injury Scale. *Journal of the American Medical Association*, 215, 277–80.

44. Civil, I.D. and Schwab C.W. (1985). The Abbreviated Injury Scale 1985 Revision: A condensed chart for clinical use. *Journal of Trauma*, 28, 87–90.

45. Civil, I.D. and Schwab, C.W. (1989). Clinical prospective injury severity scoring: when is it accurate? *Journal of Trauma*, 29, 613–14.

46. Champion, H.R., *et al.* (1980). Assesssment of injury severity: the Triage Index. *Critical Care Medicine*, 8, 201–8.

47. Champion, H.R., *et al.* (1989). A revision of the trauma score. *Journal of Trauma*, 29, 623–9.

48. Boyd, C.R., Tolson, M.A., and Copes, W.S. (1987). Evaluating trauma care. The TRISS Method. *Journal of Trauma*, 27, 370–8.

49. Champion, H.R., Sacco, W.J., and Copes W.J. (1990). A new characterization of injury severity. *Journal of Trauma*, 30, 539–46.

50. Murphy, J.G., Cayten, C.G., and Stahl, W.M. (1990). Controlling for severity of injuries in emergency medicine research. *Emergency Medicine Research*, 8, 484–9.

51. Cayten, C.G., Stahl, W.M., and Murphy, J.G. (1991). Limitations of the TRISS method for interhospital comparisions: a multi-hospital study. *Journal of Trauma*, 31, 471–82.

52. Rhee, K.J., *et al.* (1990). APACHE II scoring in the injured patient. *Critical Care Medicine*, 18, 827–830.

53. Feller, I. and Crane, K.M. (1970). National burn information exchange. *Medical Clinics of North America*, 50, 1421–36.

54. Zawacki, B.E., Azen, S.P., Imbus, S.H., and Chang, Y-T.C. (1979). Multifactorial probit analysis of mortality in burned patients. *Annals of Surgery*, 189, 1–5.

55. Lemeshow, S., *et al.* (1985). A method for predicting survival and mortality of ICU patients using objectively derived weights. *Critical Care Medicine*, 13, 519–25.

56. Teres, D., *et al.* (1987). Validation of the mortality prediction model for ICU patients. *Critical Care Medicine*, 15, 208–13.

57. Lemeshow, S., *et al.* (1988). Refining intensive care unit outcome prediction by using changing probabilities of mortality. *Critical Care Medicine*, **16**, 470–7.

58. Lemeshow, S. *et al.* (1987). A comparison of methods to predict mortality of intensive care patients. *Critical Care Medicine*, **15**, 715–22.

59. Afifi, A.A., *et al.* (1974). Prognostic indices in acute myocardial infarction complicated by shock. *American Journal of Cardiology*, **33**, 826–32.

60. Afifi, A.A., *et al.* (1971). Accumulative prognostic index for patients with barbiturate, glutethimide and meprobamate intoxication. *New England Journal of Medicine*, **285**, 1497–1503.

61. Pozen, M.W., *et al.* (1984). A predictive instrument to improve coronary care unit admission practices in acute ischaemic heart disease. *New England Journal of Medicine*, **310**, 1273–7.

62. Shoemaker, W.C. (1987). Pathophysiology, Monitoring, Outcome Prediction and Therapy of Shock States. *Critical Care Clinics*, **3**, 307–57.

63. Garden, O.J., Motyl, H., Gilmour, W.H., Utley, R.J., and Carter, D.C. (1985). Prediction of outcome following acute variceal haemorrhage. *British Journal of Surgery*, **72**, 92–5.

64. Jacobs, S., Chang, R.W.S., Lee, B., Rawaf, A., Pace, N.C., and Salam, I. (1989). Prediction of outcome in patients with acute variceal haemorrhage. *British Journal of Surgery*, **76**, 123–6.

65. Chang, R.W.S., Jacobs, S., and Lee, B. (1986). Use of Apache II severity of disease classification system to identify intensive care patients who would not benefit from total parenteral nutrition. *Lancet*, **i**, 1483–7.

66. Jacobs, S., Chang, R.W.S., and Lee, B. (1987). One year's experience with Apache II severity of disease classification system in a general ICU. *Anaesthesia*. **42**, 738–44.

67. Bion, J.F., *et al.* (1985). Validation of a prognostic score in critically ill patients undergoing transport. *British Medical Journal*, **291**, 432–4.

68. Bion, J.F., Aitchison, T.C., Edlin, S.A., and Ledingham, I. McA. (1988). Sickness scoring and response to treatment as predictors of outcome from critical illness. *Intensive Care Medicine*, **14**, 167–72.

69. Chang, R.W.S. (1989). Individual outcome prediction models for intensive care units. *Lancet*, **i**, 143–6.

70. Ridley, S., Biggam, M., and Stone, P. (1993). A cost–benefit analysis of intensive therapy. *Anaesthesia*, **48**, 14–19.

71. Chang, R.W.S., Lee, B., Jacobs, S., and Lee, B. (1989). Accuracy of decisions to withdraw therapy in critically ill patients: clinical judgement versus a computer model. *Critical Care Medicine*, **17**, 1091–7.

72. Jacobs, S., Arnold, A., Clyburn, P.A., and Willis, B.A. (1992). the Riyadh Intensive Care Program applied to a mortality analysis of a teaching hospital intensive care unit. *Anaesthesia*, **47**, 775–80.

73. Second European Consensus Conference on Intensive Care Medicine (1993, December). Predicting outcome in ICU patients. Maison de la Chimie, 28 rue Saint-Dominique, Paris 75007.

7
Quality of Life after Intensive Care

Michael Heap and Saxon A. Ridley

1. Introduction

'Quality of life' is a concept encompassing a broad range of physical and psychological characteristics that describe an individual's ability to function and derive satisfaction from doing so. Quality of life covers physical (mobility, self-care), emotional (depression, anxiety), and social functions (intimacy, social support), with role performance (work, homework), pain, and other symptoms (such as fatigue, nausea, and disease-specific symptoms). While such a broad definition is useful, quality of life measures have generally been applied to health states altered by disease and, one hopes, improved by treatment. Therefore, 'health-related quality of life' is a more appropriate term as this describes the level of well-being and satisfaction associated with an individual's life. The distinction between quality of life and the indicators of disease that are usually measured is the difference between measures of goal attainment and measures that predict goal attainment. The primary goal of health care is to provide improved survival time with an improved quality during that time. These may be considered greater achievements than the isolated correction of deranged physiological variables.

It is important to appreciate that quality of life after intensive care is only one aspect of outcome. Duration of survival may be paramount, but other concepts, such as quality of life and functional status, measure complementary facets of outcome. Functional status differs from quality of life because it considers only social roles (such as paid employment) and activities (sports and hobbies), but ignores the satisfaction derived from these roles. Functional status and other measures of an individual's activity, such as employment categories, are not strictly the same as health-related quality of life.

This chapter proposes to cover a general description of quality of life measurement. The results of quality of life assessment after intensive care will be described and the decisions and preferences regarding quality of life will be discussed. Finally, the value of intensive care units will be considered.

2. Indices of quality of life measurement

Many health-related quality of life measures are available and these cover a wide range of medical problems, of which intensive care is but one. The measurement of quality of life is difficult because there are many conceptual and methodological problems to overcome. A primary methodological consideration is whether quality of life is quantified by a profile that represents a composite measure or a summary statistic. Single measures of 'quality of life' tend to cover a single health condition (i.e. life or death), and as such are not sensitive indicators of health and well-being. However, single indicators, such as mortality and morbidity, are valuable for population monitoring, because they are the most readily available data and are sensitive to inequalities between different populations. Composite measures, covering more detailed health status and aspects of well-being, are necessary to detect and classify more subtle changes in individuals. Such composite measures divide into:

1. Health indices that summarize data from two or more components of quality of life.

2. Health profiles that measure and report several areas of quality of life; each component area may have a summary score. Health profiles may also provide a general score as a single statistic if all the components are combined.

This division into indices and profiles introduces an important controversy. Single indices of health may not capture the diversity of ideas and meaning placed on health by different individuals and therefore may be limited. Health indices and summary scores do not provide a picture of quality of life that is easily interpretable. On the other hand, a spectrum of quality of life measures described in the health profile may be easier to grasp. However, a single index summarizing health-related quality of life may be useful for policy analysis and other problems that require a unit measure. Health profiles that amalgamate their component measures can be disaggregated so that the relative contribution of each component to the total score can be individually assessed. Disaggregation is important in deciding the relationships between components and assessing the content validity of the instruments used.

There are several other methodological issues that merit consideration as these influence results. These include:

Scaling

Composite measures, either indices or profiles, imply that the individual indicators or aspects of quality of life must be weighted to allow ranking, with those having a higher score being valued as more important. In broad terms, there are three approaches to assigning weights: (1) investigator-defined; (2) relative frequencies; and (3) relative preferences. For investigator-defined weights, the investigator assigns higher scores to aspects that reflect his or her personal view of a high level of well-being or quality of life. This is the most simple and frequently used method, but the investigator assumes that he or she represents a social consensus. However, such a consensus rarely exists.[1] Also, the method of investigator-defined weights for individual aspects breaks down when the patients do not value the single aspect but a combination of attributes.

The relative frequencies method employs two techniques, factor analysis and frequency weighting. Factor analysis is a statistical technique by which items that are infrequently answered or correlate poorly, receive low weights no matter how important these items may seem in social terms.[2] Frequency weighting is based on the cumulative scaling principle that explores the extent to which attributes can be ordered in a sequence along a single continuum and so given a scale.[3] Unfortunately, large populations are required to form a representative sample of possible sequences. There is also the theoretical objection that the identification of a scale does not exclude the possibility that other ideas are present or are being measured.[4]

The relative preference methods involve assessing the relative desirability of different health states using specified rules. Selected health states are ranked according to how much better or worse each appears by comparison to the others.[5]

Aggregation

Aggregation and use of individual components of a score have been outlined above. Furthermore, summing disparate dimensions may reduce the sensitivity because contradictory trends for different aspects of quality of life are disguised. There are no firmly held views about which is the best aggregation method; however, quality adjusted life years (QALYs) is one summary score that is widely used.[6]

Reliability and stability

In any research tool these two ideas are important. Reliability estimates the proportion of the observed variation that can be considered true as opposed to random error. The minimum error of reliability differs according to the type of study being conducted. Ware[7] has suggested that reliability coefficients of above 0.9 are required for comparisons between individuals, whereas for comparison between populations the coefficients may be lower (0.5–0.7). Reliability of quality of life measures may be calculated using internal consistency. This involves measuring the degree of agreement between two components quantifying the same aspect of quality of life. Reliability can also be assessed using sequential testing of the same subjects with the same questionnaire.

The stability reflects the fluctuation in scores over longer periods, usually six months or more.[8] As with reliability, stability measures the degree of true, as opposed to random, error.

Validity

The validity of a measurement is the extent to which it appropriately measures that which it is intended to measure. For quality of life, this is difficult because the instruments are measuring an inherently subjective phenomenon. Usually in science, validity involves comparison of the measurement with a 'gold standard'. Unfortunately, for most quality of life measures no such gold standard exists and indirect approaches to the validation of the measurement are required. Furthermore, there are many different types of validity (concurrent, convergent, predictive, or construct), with many different empirical approaches for measuring such validity.[7]

Considering these issues Moriyama[9] has identified six desirable properties for evaluating health-related quality of life indices, irrespective of how the index is derived. These include:

1. It should be meaningful and understandable.

2. It should be sensitive to the variations in the phenomena being measured.

3. The assumptions underlying the index should be theoretically justifiable and intuitively reasonable.

4. It should consist of clearly defined component parts.

5. Each component should make an independent contribution to the measurement.

6. The index should be derivable from data that are available or possible to obtain.

Therefore, an adequate assessment of health-related quality of life should include an explicit statement of the individual's own evaluation of his or her own health status. These evaluations are required for estimates of reliability and validity. The individual's evaluation of quality of life should be assessed using a standardized questionnaire so that comparable information is elicited. This will provide policy-makers with more useful information than by using untested non-standardized instruments.

After specific medical therapies, both general health and disease-specific measures of quality of life are important. The relative value of disease-specific measures versus general measures of health depends on the purpose of the research. For example, disease-specific measures are likely to show a statistically significant difference between ineffective and effective therapies. However, such disease-specific measures may offer little information concerning which therapy was more toxic, if toxicity was manifested in an organ system not involved in the primary disease. Under these circumstances, a measure of general health would be more valuable. However, the disadvantage of general health measures is that they may be too insensitive because they

Table 7.1 Practical considerations for selecting a measure of health-related quality of life

---

1. Standardized or non-standardized instruments
   • Identification of real differences among selected clinical problems
   • Resource requirement/time and effort

2. Acceptability
   • Previous experiences in the clinical applications
   • Respondent burden—the 'unhealthy' respondent
   • Interviewer burden

3. Method of administration
   • Direct observation
   • Face-to-face interview
   • Telephone interview
   • Self-administered questionnaire
   • Proxy respondence

4. Length and cost of administration
   • Other components of interview or questionnaire
   • Completion rates and quality of data

5. Methods of analysis and complexity of scoring
   • Aggregation or disaggregation into component parts

6. Usefulness to decision-makers
   • Degree of certainty on value

---

include items not relevant to the particular disease. Because of the diversity of pathophysiology treated in intensive care, many disease-specific measures would be required. Therefore, for intensive care, general measures of health are likely to be the most appropriate.

Finally, there are some practical considerations to take into account when selecting a measure of health-related quality of life (Table 7.1). Developing an instrument for a specific application, such as intensive care, may initially seem attractive because of the apparent uniqueness and complexity of the clinical problem. However, a unique instrument cannot be used outside its specific application and so comparisons with other health care programmes are not possible. Furthermore, developing a new health-related quality of life measure requires substantial time, effort, and careful thought. An alternative to developing a new instrument is to use a standardized general health questionnaire. Such an approach offers a global measurement of quality of life but also allows scope for careful assessment of specific relevant areas.

Acceptability refers to the ease with which an instrument can be used in any particular setting and is based on previous experience of the instrument. Acceptability is concerned with how well the instrument satisfies the research needs, available resources, and the burden that answering the questionnaire places on the respondent, both in terms of time and psychological stress. The length of response time may differ significantly because of personal characteristics of the respondent such as age, education, and health status. Furthermore, patients on certain sedative agents may have impaired memory and cognitive function.

The different methods of administration vary significantly in their costs and the participation required from both researcher and respondent. Some instruments have been specifically developed as self-completed postal questionnaires and these are the simplest to administer. However, research suggests that certain types of therapy, for example knee replacements, cannot be adequately assessed by postal surveys alone.[10]

3. Quality of life assessment

As with other areas of medicine, interest in health-related quality of life after discharge from intensive care units (ICUs) has only recently become a topic for consideration, research, and evaluation. A few studies [11-14] have reported quality of life using only broad descriptive terms that did not critically assess aspects of function and satisfaction. More recently, specific quality of life measures have been developed and applied to ICU survivors in projects whose main aim was quality of life assessment.[15,16]

However, whichever type of quality of life assessment is used, patients admitted to the ICU are not a random selection from the general population. Critically ill patients are admitted with a heterogeneous range of diagnoses and are bound together only by their life-threatening physiological disturbance. Their physical impairment generally stems from pre-existing conditions and as a result their spectrum of pre-morbid quality of life is generally less than that expected in normal individuals. Goldstein *et al.*[17] examined the physical activities of ICU patients before acute illness. In a patient population of 2300, 12 per cent of patients' activities were severely limited before admission; only 41 per cent of the patients were previously able to undertake moderate or heavy activity, while the remainder were either involved in sedentary or mild activity. Fifteen per cent of patients, who were below retirement age, were registered disabled; this was the same proportion as those without work. In the UK, the pre-admission quality of life for 17 per cent of critically ill patients was poor[16]. Patients placed their pre-morbid quality of life in the three lowest of Rosser's Disability Categories (i.e. V–VII). This represents severe physical and social impairment. With such distribution of poor pre-existing functional and employment status, the scope for improvement under medical intervention may be poor, especially if such impairment is long-standing.

Goldstein *et al.*[17] reported that over 70 per cent of previously active patients were capable of only mild or sedentary activity after discharge. Patients who were limited to sedentary activity remained about the same. There was improvement in the small number of patients who were severely limited on admission (n = 66) after medical intensive care. However, these changes in quality of life could be attributed to the disease process rather than the effectiveness and quality of care received in the ICU.

The main aim of intensive care is to save life rather than improve it. While improvements are welcome, they are unlikely to be comparable with those following joint replacement, effective arthritis treatment, and appropriate cancer therapy. Furthermore, intensive care management may only be required for a brief period while the acute physiological disturbances are corrected. The distribution of duration of admission to the ICU is heavily skewed with most patients being treated for only a few days.[18] These patients' quality of life after hospital discharge is unlikely to be significantly influenced by their brief treatment on intensive care.

However, a few intensive care patients remain in ICUs for extended periods of time. Such patients have both reduced survival and significant decreases in their quality of life. For example, Spicher and White[19] classified the functional status of 250 long-term ventilated patients into three very broad groups. The mean duration of admission for these patients was 31 days but the range extended from 10 to over 300 days. Spicher noted that age and functional status (i.e. the activities of daily living) were predictors of survival. Forty per cent of survivors were discharged to nursing homes, and another 33 per cent were confined to their own homes. Zaren and Hedstrand[13] classified the health status of 980 critically ill patients. Seventy per cent of survivors, who were treated in ICUs for over one week, lived independently afterwards. If admission was shorter, 90 per cent of the survivors were subsequently independent.

Zaren and Hedstrand confirmed the effect of pre-morbid functional ability on post-discharge status; 88 per cent of patients, who lived independently in the three months before admission, returned to live independently one year after admission. As in Goldstein *et al.*'s study, Zaren and Hedstrand found that the quality of life for a few patients with pre-existing severe limitation improved significantly.

However, such improvements may have been a floor effect. Patients with a very poor quality of life who obtained minimum rankings before treatment may not have any scope to register any further deterioration. Unfortunately, few details were given about such severely limited patients. Zaren and Hedstrand also noted that there was little improvement in quality of life after six months. This may be an appropriate time to assess quality of life as the effects of recall bias and other sociodemographic factors will be minimized.

Trauma victims generally regained a good level of functional recovery, with most caring for themselves. The encouraging results for trauma victims have been supported by work from Kivioja *et al.*[20] They reported that 72 per cent of patients admitted with severe trauma were still working 5 to 20 years after their accident.

Quality of life after intensive care has been assessed using Rosser's disability categories.[16] Quality of life assessment before and after critical illness was assessed using a self-completed postal questionnaire distributed to patients between one and three years after discharge. Of all the diagnostic categories only the trauma victims ($n = 26$) reported significant decreases in their quality of life. While trauma victims may benefit most from intensive care management in terms of survival, it is particularly interesting that these patients suffered significant decreases in their quality of life. Most of the trauma victims were young (median age 20) and so their expectation of life may be assumed to be greater than an older population.

Thiagarajan *et al.*[21] examined the quality of life of trauma victims more closely. They used the Nottingham Health Profile,[22] a general health profile, and the Perceived Quality of Life Scale, a utility covering general health, but one that was specifically designed for use in intensive care.[15] The trauma victims reported significant decreases in their quality of life in relation to their health, happiness, ability to think, pursue leisure activities, their income, and their employment. Their mean perceived quality of life scale decreased by 13 per cent (95 per cent confidence limits 7.5–19.5 per cent), but 62 per cent of survivors experienced severe social disability and modest or severe impairment at work. The Nottingham Health Profile identified major changes in the psychological aspects of quality of life, namely, energy and emotional reactions. Comparisons of quality of life after simple fractures[23] suggest a similar distribution of problems as detected by the Nottingham Health Profile after severe life-threatening trauma. Such prominent psychological problems in the two studies may suggest that it is not necessarily the severity of the trauma alone that influences its impact on quality of life. Whatever the precise mechanism, further rehabilitation concentrating on less physical attributes of the injury may improve quality of life and so achieve a more satisfactory result than simply increased survival.

Mundt *et al.*[24] studied the employment and functional status of 887 patients; functional status was divided into psychological, physical, and social. Their assessment of quality of life was not scaled, only a direction of the change was recorded. The physical variables reflected only one significant decrease, namely, the ability to do housework. However, for the psychological variables, there was a significant decrease in the ability to concentrate and think clearly. All of the social variables were associated with significant changes in that the patients were less involved in leisure activities and had less contact with friends, but more contact with family members. Again, this study emphasized the importance of the psychological and social deteriorations compared to physical changes.

In summary, quality of life after intensive care varies and is not the same as functional activity. This is best illustrated by trauma victims who regain a high level of functional activity but suffer serious deteriorations in the psychological aspects of the quality of life. Patients admitted to ICUs have a poorer pre-morbid quality of life than expected. Although many patients regain their pre-morbid quality of life, some suffer significant decreases, especially if their intensive care management was prolonged.

4. Decisions and preferences

Quality of life measures significantly influence decisions to initiate, with-hold, or withdraw intensive care. However, their influence has been largely unquantified and there is confusion about which aspects of quality of life are important and from whose standpoint they should be considered.

It is helpful to consider four situations where quality of life is most likely to influence decision-making. First, there is the patient whose quality of life prior to critical illness is very poor. Intensive care physicians see only a minority of these patients as many are not referred for intensive care. The second scenario includes patients with a very poor quality of life as a result of critical illness. This occurs most commonly following cerebral trauma or hypoxia. Patients with no hope of survival form the third group and pose less of an ethical dilemma. However, their quality of life may influence the timing of treatment withdrawal. The last situation is characterized by patients where both the prognosis and predicted quality of life appear poor, but can not be clearly defined or quantified. Such uncertainty may lead to greater scrutiny of patients' quality of life.

There is no doubt that patients' quality of life does influence clinicians. Patients with pre-existing dementia are seldom admitted to ICUs in the UK. In an American study of DNRs (do-not-resuscitate orders), 33 per cent of DNRs were made because of an unacceptable quality of life.[25] However, theoretically, it may be inappropriate for clinicians to make decisions based on another person's quality of life.

First, only the patient can gauge the satisfaction that he or she gains from life. What may be an intolerable burden for one person may be easily accepted by another. Thus, objective measures, such as ability to return to work and to live independently, may correlate only moderately with more subjective measures of quality of life, such as the patient's perceived satisfaction with life.[15] In particular, older people's satisfaction with life may be well maintained despite significant reductions in function.[26]

Second, the widespread belief that physicians can accurately predict patients' preferences concerning intensive care is false.[27] Uhlmann *et al.* found that, in most cases, physicians were no better at predicting the patients' preferences than chance alone.[28] Intensive care nurses are also unable to predict the desires of survivors to return to intensive care if the need arose.[29,30] Physicians and nurses tend to overestimate the importance of quality of life and to err on the side of withholding treatment.[27-30]

Finally, patient autonomy suggests that irrespective of physicians' estimates of quality of life or perceived preferences, the patients should decide on these important aspects of their treatment. Paternalistic decisions made by clinicians on behalf of their patients may be unjust as well as inaccurate. They may also be influenced by other factors such as the age, religious beliefs, cultural, and medical background of the clinicians themselves.

A more logical and just solution may involve the patients themselves deciding how their quality of life will influence the decision to withhold or withdraw intensive care. There are, however, a number of questions that need to be addressed in relation to this.

1. Are patients' preferences influenced by their quality of life?

2. Do patients wish to decide for themselves?

3. Are patients in a position to make a rational decision?

Several studies have shown that a proportion of patients would not want intensive care under certain circumstances, such as persistent coma, dementia, or the absence of any hope of recovery.[31-35] For these patients, quality of life obviously influences their treatment preferences. The most important determining factors are cognitive ability, dependence on relatives, chronic pain, and prognosis.[36,37] However, one striking feature of many of these studies is that there are also subgroups of patients who hold more extreme views in which the quality of life has little or no importance. One study found that 30 per cent of patients always wanted artificial ventilation in the event of critical illness, irrespective of prognosis and quality of life, whereas 14 per cent never wanted treatment.[36] Patients' preferences for intensive care are thus extremely variable. While many are influenced by significant reductions in quality of life, others prefer survival at any cost.

Some patients do not wish to decide about their treatment, even if given the choice. Forty per cent of an elderly British sample wanted to decide about initiation of artificial ventilation themselves. Twenty-five per cent, while wanting to be fully informed, wished to leave the decision to medical staff, and 29 per cent preferred not to know anything about it. If they were to become incompetent, 76 per cent were happy to leave the decision about artificial ventilation to medical staff, either alone, or with the help of relatives, while 24 per cent wanted to use some form of advance directive.[36] These figures suggest that most elderly patients are confident of the ability of doctors and nurses to look after their best interests.

Critical illness imposes severe limitations on the validity of patient autonomy, which, ideally, requires patients to be mentally competent (i.e. free from the effect of psychotropic drugs and neurological manifestations of critical illness) and fully informed. Fisher and Raper[38] have pointed out that the apparently competent critically ill patient may not be entirely rational, and that patients who initially refuse treatment may later change their minds. However, it may be difficult to distinguish between an irrational patient (in the eyes of the medical staff) and an incompetent patient exercising his autonomy. Furthermore, even competent patients may not truly understand the complexities of intensive care, the uncertainties of outcome prediction, and so the balance between burden and benefit.

For these reasons, the idea that patients should make their own decisions about intensive care is frequently impractical. For example, where the validity of a patient's treatment refusal is in doubt, it would be entirely appropriate to continue treatment. It is always safest to err on the side of preserving life. Withdrawal of treatment is more difficult and there is rarely a chance for second thoughts. Clinicians must be entirely satisfied that withdrawal is in the best interests of their patient. They must avoid imposing their own values and seek instead to determine those of the patient. The difficulties with this have already been discussed. Unfortunately, no patient characteristics, including age, have been found consistently to correlate with treatment preferences. Some help may come from patients' relatives and from the use of advance directives.

Relatives are better at predicting patients' preferences than primary care physicians, although the proportion of discordant responses is still high.[27] They are less likely than physicians to withhold treatment that the patient would in fact want, and so may contribute to a more balanced assessment.[28] However, relatives may disagree with physicians for less constructive reasons, such as guilt, denial, and fear. Osborne has emphasized the value of counselling in these situations and more time may be required before consensus is reached.[39,40] Making decisions on behalf of an incompetent relative has been likened to having to choose between acting as torturer or executioner. Fisher and Raper feel that in their experience few Australians wish to take on such a role. They therefore 'seek concurrence on a medical management plan and never seek permission to change to alternative treatment'.[41] American physicians appear to be less authoritarian.[42]

Advance directives (living wills) may offer an alternative source of guidance when making decisions about incompetent patients (see Chapter 5). The advance directive has become increasingly popular, particularly in America, but it has several limitations. Patients' views on future events, while still in good health, may not correspond to their views when faced with a life-threatening illness. The clinical situations covered by advance directives tend to be limited and clear-cut, which contrast with the complex clinical pictures in the ICU. In fact, advance directives have been dismissed as irrelevant as they merely reflect accepted best medical practice—the avoidance of unnecessary suffering and prolongation of dying.[38,43] However, this perspective ignores the variable and unpredictable nature of patients' preferences. For example, the patient who would refuse artificial ventilation if he or she were to develop permanent cognitive impairment can only be distinguished from one who prefers survival at any cost, by the use of some form of advance planning. The advance directive may have a useful role, but requires improvement. A working party report suggested combining the directive with an arrangement for third-party decision-making, for example a durable power of attorney for health care.[44] If detailed discussions have taken place between patient and proxy, this provides probably the most efficient method of substituted judgement and has the additional advantage of flexibility. However, such a combination is rarely used at present.[40]

When decisions to withhold or withdraw intensive care are based on quality of life considerations, there are compelling reasons to ensure that the patient is fully involved whenever possible. In the UK, the introduction of this principle into clinical practice has already begun.[45,46] Nevertheless, the doctor's role as patient's advocate is often unavoidable as patients may be reluctant to or incapable of participating in decision-making. This should not be used as an excuse for paternalism, but undertaken in the light of our knowledge of the unpredictable and variable nature of both patients' life satisfaction and treatment preferences.

5. Value of intensive care

The value of intensive care is very difficult to define; as discussed earlier, it can be measured in terms of health-related quality of life changes after treatment. However, as already mentioned, the main aim of intensive care is to save life as opposed to actively improve it. Quality of life is undoubtedly important and should contribute to the valuation of intensive care's worth but it is not the principal component. Furthermore, the question arises, should the value of intensive care be estimated in economic terms, namely cost, or should it be valued in more human terms? If human terms are chosen, how is life valued? If a valuation of intensive care is required, then intensive care must be compared to another standard so that it can be ranked and compared with other health interventions. Such considerations make the valuation of intensive care difficult.

The value of intensive care may be gauged by how well it achieves its primary goal, namely its ability to save lives. Unfortunately, intensive care services have evolved over the last 30 years as techniques in medicine and surgery have advanced. During this time, no controlled trials compared intensive care to other levels of care elsewhere in the hospital. Today, intensive care has advanced to such a level that it may be considered unethical to randomly assign patients to receive either intensive care or other care on a general ward. Therefore, intensive care is assumed to be more effective than other forms of care at saving critically ill patients' lives but this has not been scientifically proved.

Survival after intensive care varies. There are groups of patients who do benefit from intensive care and for these patients, intensive care can be considered valuable. For example, the survival of trauma victims is generally good providing they survive their initial injury.[47] However there are certain subgroups of critically ill patients who suffer particularly high mortality. Such groups of patients include those with renal failure[48] and sepsis;[49] unfortunately, it is these patients who require the technological support available in the intensive care unit if they are to have any chance of survival.

It is necessary to examine the survival of all intensive care patients rather than specific subsets. It could be argued that as intensive care's main aim is to save life the best result that can be obtained is a return of normal life expectancy for long-term survivors. However, as alluded to in Goldstein *et al.*'s study,[17] patients admitted to intensive care units are not a random selection of the normal population. There is a preponderance of patients with chronic disease or reduced physiological reserve, two factors that influence survival.[50,51] With these caveats, long-term survival after intensive care may provide some estimate of its value. It is not clear what the optimum follow-up from intensive care should be. Zaren and Bergstrom[52] suggested that the survival of intensive care patients paralleled that of the general population after six months. In a smaller study LeGall *et al.*[53] appeared to confirm that only short follow-up times were needed. However, in a study of over 1000 critically ill patients, their survival curve did not parallel that of an age-and sex-matched general population until the start of the fourth year (Fig. 7.1).[54]

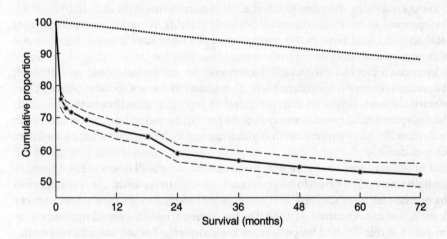

Fig. 7.1 Survival curve for ICU patients (solid line) and an age and sex-matched population (broken line). The 95 per cent confidence limits for ICU patients are shown (after Ridley and Plenderleith).[54]

Patients dying more rapidly than expected may not appear to have benefited from intensive care. However, at the time of their admission, they benefit greatly from the levels of observation and monitoring available in the ICU and at that stage their prognosis is unknown.

Accepting that some patients die rapidly after intensive care and that certain groups of patients have poor prognoses, can the present use of intensive care be improved? Intensive care can be broadly defined as a service for patients with potentially recoverable conditions who can benefit from more detailed observation and treatment that are generally unavailable in the general wards and departments. However, once admitted to an ICU, it can be difficult to prove how patients benefit during their stay. Ron *et al.*[55] cleverly bypassed the ethical considerations of randomizing patients to receive or not to receive intensive care. By matching survivors and fatalities (in a 3:1 ration), they analysed the mortality rate in several patient groups divided according to severity of illness, stability, and whether the patients were treated in the ICU or general hospital ward. Only 'unstable moderately ill' patients, who accounted for only 4 per cent of all hospital admissions, had reduced mortality (4 vs. 18 per cent) when admitted directly to intensive care. In the US, Knaus *et al.*[56] reported that 20 per cent of ICU admissions were for observation and monitoring but only a fraction of these required further intensive care measures. In the UK, a recent study suggested that 40 per cent of patients treated in the ICU had a risk of hospital mortality of less than 10 per cent.[57] These results suggest that many patients do not directly benefit from intensive care intervention and therefore this type of care for such patients was of little value. However, as intensive care has evolved over the years, there is now a large gulf between the care available in the ICU and the general ward. A recent study by the Royal College of Anaesthetists[58] found that the ICU was supported by a high dependency unit (HDU) in only 39 hospitals. The HDU could admit patients who are potentially unstable but who require only observation and monitoring.

Intensive care is undoubtedly expensive; its economic value, in terms of resource consumption, is high. Bams and Miranda[14] showed that in the course of critical illness, only a sixth of the total hospital stay was spent in the ICU, but that 52 per cent of costs associated with the illness were incurred on intensive care. Loes *et al.*[11] estimated that intensive care management accounted for 32 per cent of the total cost of any illness and other studies[59-61] confirm that intensive care costs represent between 30 and 50 per cent of total hospital costs. However, intensive care is not necessarily more expensive than other high-technology and labour-dependent health care programmes. A table indicating costs per QALY for various health care programmes is shown in Table 7.2.[62] The cost of treating survivors of critical illness is high, lying between those of heart transplantation and haemodialysis. Therefore, the value of intensive care in terms of resources of consumption is high, but not necessarily higher than that of other hospital programmes.

Table 7.2 Cost per QALY rankings (after Ridley *et al.*)[62]

Treatment	Cost/QALY
Pacemaker implantation	£830
Hip replacement	£890
CAVG (moderate angina, left main disease)	£1580
Kidney transplant	£3560
Heart transplant	£6070
Respiratory or cardiovascular critical illness	£7500
Haemodialysis at home	£13 070
Haemodialysis in hospital	£16 630

CAVG: Coronary Artery Vein Grafts.
QALY: Quality adjusted life year (after Kind *et al.*, note 6)

Improvements in the value of intensive care pose a difficult dilemma. The most important area is probably patient selection. If patients, who are presently treated in the ICU (for observation and monitoring), can be treated elsewhere, such as a high dependency unit (HDU), the cost of treatment will be lower. Unfortunately, some patients, by nature of the pathophysiological insult and their physiological reserve, are unlikely to survive critical illness. It is important to identify such patients and closely monitor their progress so that intensive care does not prolong their death. The effect of increasing mortality in the ICU on the cost per survivor is illustrated in Fig. 7.2.[54] Death in the ICU is a tragedy both in human terms, and because of the high cost of treatment in economic terms. A high mortality rate in the ICU and in the early discharge phase will raise the costs and make each survivor more expensive. The increase in cost per survivor is exponential and therefore careful patient selection and appropriate application of intensive care once the patient is admitted may yield small reductions in mortality, but produce significant financial savings. Such an approach will improve the value, in fiscal terms, of intensive care.

6. Conclusion

Quality of life measurement is an important aspect when considering the success of medical treatment. However, following the intensive care management of critical illness, quality of life changes may be of secondary importance and are dependent on the pathophysiology involved rather than the treatment received. Methods for quality of life assessment are well established but have been infrequently applied to intensive care. The results of studies suggest that the pre-morbid quality of life of critically ill patients is poorer than expected and the changes following treatment depend on the type and duration of illness.

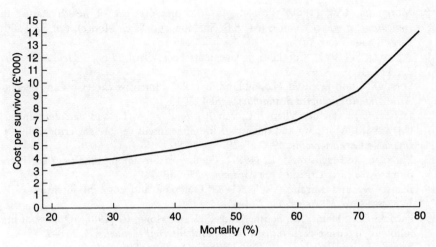

Fig. 7.2 The effect of increasing mortality on cost per survivor (after Ridley and Plenderleith).[54]

Unless the patients have been specifically questioned, it can be difficult to make decisions about changes in the direction of intensive care management as patient preferences vary widely. The value of intensive care involves more than simple cost minimization; it includes support facilities such as high dependency units and prognosis prediction.

Notes

1. Torrance, G.W. (1976). Social preference for health states: An empirical evaluation of three measurement techniques. *Socioeconomic Plan Science*, **10**, 128–36.
2. Kaplan, R.M., Bush, J.W., and Berry, C.C. (1976). Health status: Types of validity and the Index of Well-Being. *Health Services Research*, **11**, 478–507.
3. Guttman, L.A. (1944). A basis for scaling qualitative data. *American Sociology Review*, **91**, 139–50.
4. Williams, R. (1983). Disability as a health indicator. In *Health Indicators* , (ed. A.J. Culyer), pp. 150–64. Martin Robertson, Oxford.
5. Torrance, G.W. (1986). Measurement of health state utilities for economic appraisal. *Journal of Health Economics*, **5**, 1–30.
6. Kind, P., Rosser, R., and Williams, A. (1982). Valuation of quality of life: some psychometric evidence. In *The value of life and safety*, (ed. M.W. Jones-Lee), pp. 159–70. North Holland, Amsterdam.
7. Ware, J.E. (1984). Methodological considerations in selection of health status assessment procedures. In *Assessment of quality of life in clinical trials of cardiovascular therapies*, (ed. N.K. Wenger *et al.*), pp. 87–111. Le Jacq, New York.
8. Nunnally, J.C. (1978). *Psychometric theory*. McGraw-Hill, New York.

9. Moriyama, I.W. (1968). Problems in the measurement of health status. In *Indicators of social change*, (ed. E.B. Sheldon and W.E. Moore), pp. 573–600. Russell Sage, New York.

10. Brewster, S. (1991). Can knee replacements be assessed by post? *Health Trends*, **23**, 113–4.

11. Loes, O., Smith-Erichsen, N., and Lind, B. (1987). Intensive care: Cost and benefit. *Acta Anaesthesiologica Scandinavica*, **S84**, 3–19.

12. Jacobs, C.J., van der Vliet, J.A., van Roozendaal, M.T., and van der Linden, C.J. (1988). Mortality and quality of life after intensive care for critical illness. *Intensive Care Medicine*, **14**, 217–20.

13. Zaren, B. and Hedstrand, U. (1987). Quality of life among long-term survivors of intensive care. *Critical Care Medicine*, **15**, 743–7.

14. Bams, J.L. and Miranda, D.R. (1985).Outcome and costs of intensive care. *Intensive Care Medicine*, **11**, 234–41.

15. Patrick, D.L., Danis, M., Southerland, L.I., and Hong, G. (1988). Quality of life following intensive care. *Journal of General Internal Medicine*, **3**, 218–23.

16. Ridley, S. and Wallace, P.G.M. (1990). Quality of life after intensive care. *Anaesthesia*, **45**, 808–13.

17. Goldstein, R.L., Campion, E.W., Thibault, G.E., Mulley, A.G., and Skinner, E. (1986). Functional outcomes following medical intensice care. *Critical Care Medicine*, **14**, 783–8.

18. Cohen, A., Bodenham, A., and Webster, N. (1993). A review of 2000 consecutive ICU admissions. *Anaesthesia*, **48**, 106–10.

19. Spicher, J.E. and White, D.P. (1987). Outcome and function following prolonged mechanical ventilation. *Archives of Internal Medicine*, **147**, 421–5.

20. Kivioja, A.H., Myllynen, P.J., and Rokkanen, P.U. (1990). Is the treatment of the most severe multiply injured patients worth the effort? A follow up examination 5 to 20 years after severe multiple injury. *Journal of Trauma*, **30**, 480–3.

21. Thiagarajan, J., Taylor, P., Hogbin, E., and Ridley, S. (1994). Quality of life after multiple trauma requiring intensive care. *Anaesthesia*, **49**, 211–18.

22. Hunt, S., McEwen, J., and McKenna, S. (1985). Measuring health status: a new tool for clinicians and epidemiologists. *Journal of the Royal College of General Practitioners*, **35**, 185–8.

23. McKenna, S., McEwen, J., and Hunt, S. (1984). Changes in perceived health of patients recovering from fractures. *Public Health*, **88**, 97–102.

24. Mundt, D.J., Gage, R.W., Lemeshow, S., Pastides, H., Teres, D., and Avrunin, J.S. (1989). Intensive care unit patient follow-up. *Archives of Internal Medicine*, **149**, 68–72.

25. Gleeson, K. and Wise, S. (1990). The do-not-resuscitate order. Still too little too late. *Archives of Internal Medicine*, **150**, 1057–60.

26. Sage, W.M., Rosenthal, M.H., and Silverman, J.F. (1986). Is intensive care worth it? An assessment of input and outcome for the critically ill. *Critical Care Medicine*, **14**, 777–82.

27. Seckler, A.B., Meier, D.E., Mulvihill, M., and Cammer Paris, B.E. (1991). Substituted judgement: How accurate are proxy predictions? *Annals of Internal Medicine*, **115**, 92–8.

28. Uhlmann, R.F., Pearlman, R.A., and Cain, K.C. (1988). Physicians' and spouses'

predictions of elderly patients' resuscitation preferences. *Journal of Gerontology*, **43**, 115–21.

29. Danis, M., Jarr, S.L., Southerland, L.I., Nocella, R.S., and Patrick, D.L. (1987). A comparison of patient, family, and nurse evaluations of the usefulness of intensive care. *Critical Care Medicine*, **15**, 138–43.

30. Boyle, M., Kwasha, D., and Morris, R.W. (1991). Do intensive care nurses consider intensive care less useful than their patients or patient's family? *Confederation of Australian Critical Care Nurses Journal* **4**, 22–7.

31. Danis, M., *et al.* (1991). A prospective study of advance directives for life-sustaining care. *New England Journal of Medicine*, **324**, 882–8.

32. Frankl, D., Oye, R.K., and Bellamy, P.E. (1989). Attitudes of hospitalized patients toward life support: a survey of 200 medical inpatients. *American Journal of Medicine*, **86**, 645–8.

33. Emanuel, L.L., Barry, M.J., Stoeckle, J.D., Ettelson, L.M., and Emanuel, E.J. (1991). Advance directives for medical care—a case for greater use. *New England Journal of Medicine*, **324**, 889–95.

34. Lo, B., Mcleod, G.A., and Saika, G. (1986). Patient attitudes to discussing life-sustaining treatment. *Archives of Internal Medicine*, **146**, 1613–5.

35. Danis, M., Patrick, D.L., Southerland, L.I., and Green, M.L. (1988). Patients' and families' preferences for medical intensive care. *Journal of the American Medical Association*, **260**, 797–802.

36. Heap, M.J., Munglani, R., Klinck, J.R., and Males, A.G. (1993). Elderly patients' preferences concerning life-support treatment. *Anaesthesia*, **48**, 1027–33.

37. Zweibel, N.R. and Cassel, C.K. (1989). Treatment choices at the end of life: a comparison of decisions by older patients and their physician-selected proxies. *Gerontologist*, **29**, 615–21.

38. Fisher, M.M. and Raper, R.F. (1990). Withdrawing and withholding treatment in intensive care. Part 1. Social and ethical dimensions. *Medical Journal of Australia*, **153**, 217–20.

39. Osborne, M.L. (1992). Physician decisions regarding life support in the intensive care unit. *Chest*, **101**, 217–24.

40. Smedira, N.G., *et al.* (1990). Withholding and withdrawal of life support from the critically ill. *New England Journal of Medicine*, **322**, 309–15.

41. Fisher, M.M. and Raper, R.F. (1990). Withdrawing and withholding treatment in intensive care. Part 3. Practical aspects. *Medical Journal of Australia*, **153**, 222–5.

42. Miller, D.K., Coe, R.M., and Hyers, T.M. (1992). Achieving consensus on withdrawing or withholding care for critically ill patients. *Journal of General Internal Medicine*, **7**, 475–80.

43. Orlowski, J.P. (1986). Ethical principles in critical care medicine. *Critical Care Clinics*, **2**, 13–25.

44. Age Concern Institute of Gerontology and the Centre of Medical Law and Ethics, King's College, London (1988). *The living will: Consent to treatment at the end of life. A working party report.* Edward Arnold, London.

45. Broadway, P.J., Forsyth, D.R., and Park, G.R. (1993). The do-not-resuscitate order in the intensive care unit. *British Journal of Intensive Care*, **3**, 318–22.

46. Doyal, L. and Wilsher, D. (1993). Withholding cardiopulmonary resuscitation: proposals for formal guidelines. *British Medical Journal*, **306**, 1593–6.

47. Goins, W.A., Reynolds, H.N., Nyanjom, D., and Dunham, M. (1991). Outcome following prolonged intensive care unit stay in multiple trauma patients. *Critical Care Medicine*, 19, 339–45.
48. Maher, E.R., *et al.* (1989). Prognosis of critically ill patients with acute renal failure: APACHE II score and other predictive factors. *Quarterly Journal of Medicine*, 72, 256–66.
49. Knaus, W.A., Draper, E.A., Wagner, D.P., Zimmerman, J.E. (1985). Prognosis in acute organ-system failure. *Annals of Surgery*, 202, 685–93.
50. Tran, D.D., Groeneveld, A.B.J., van der Meulen, J., Nauta, J.J.P., van Schundel, R.J., and Thus, L.G. (1990). Age, chronic disease, sepsis, organ system failure and mortality in a medical intensive care unit. *Critical Care Medicine*, 18, 474–9.
51. Knaus, W.A., Draper, E.A., Wagner, D.P., and Zimmerman, J.E. (1985). APACHE II: A severity of disease classification system. *Critical Care Medicine*, 13, 818–29.
52. Zaren, B., and Bergstrom, R. (1989). Survival compared to the general population and changes in health status among intensive care patients. *Acta Anaesthesiologica Scandinavica*, 33, 6–12.
53. Le Gall, J., Brun-Buisson, C., Trunet, P., Latournerie, J., Chantereau, S., and Rapin, M. (1982). Influence of age, previous health status, and severity of acute illness on outcome from intensive care. *Critical Care Medicine*, 10, 575–7.
54. Ridley, S. and Plenderleith, L. (1994). Survival after intensive care. Comparison with a normal matched population as an indicator of effectiveness. *Anaesthesia*, 49, 933–5.
55. Ron, A., Aronne, L.J., Kalb, P.E., Santini, D., and Charlson, M.E. (1989). The therapeutic efficacy of critical care units. Identifying subgroups of patients who benefit. *Archives of Internal Medicine*, 149, 338–41.
56. Knaus, W.A., *et al.* (1982). Evaluating outcome for intensive care; a preliminary multi-hospital comparison. *Critical Care Medicine*, 10, 491–6.
57. Kilpatrick, A., Ridley, S., and Plenderleith, L. (1994). A changing role for intensive therapy: Is there a case for high dependency care? *Anaesthesia*, 49, 666–70.
58. Stoddard, J. (1993). *National ITU audit 1992/1993*. The Royal College of Anaesthetists, London.
59. Parno, J.R., Teres, D., Lemeshow, S., Brown, R.V. (1982). Hospital charges and long-term survival of ICU versus non-ICU patients. *Critical Care Medicine*, 10, 569–74.
60. Civetta, J.M. and Hudson-Civetta, J.A. (1985). Maintaining quality of care while reducing charges in the ICU. *Annals of Surgery*, 202, 524–32.
61. Havill, J.H., Walker, L., and Sceats, J.E. (1989). Three hundred admissions to the Waikato Hospital intensive therapy unit—survival, costs and quality of life after 2 years. *New Zealand Medical Journal*, 102, 179–81.
62. Ridley, S., Biggam, M., and Stone, P. (1994). A cost–utility analysis of intensive therapy. *Anaesthesia*, 49, 192–6.

N.S. Morton

The ethical issues encountered in paediatric and neonatal intensive care encompass many of the subjects covered in this book but there are aspects that are peculiar to the care of children where decision-making is often, of necessity, by proxy. Of particular current concern are selection for intensive care, consent to treatment, witholding or withdrawing intensive care, diagnosis of brain death, organ donation, and research on children. These issues are tackled every day by clinicians but advances in technology, pharmacology, understanding of diseases, financial constraints, cultural variability, and legal limitations all influence the approach to individual cases.

1. Neonatal intensive care

Rapid advances in neonatology have pushed down the limits of satisfactory viability to around 24 weeks of gestation, with occasional individuals surviving below this age. This has led to a reconsideration of the legal limit for termination of pregnancy, re-evaluation of selection criteria for offering neonatal intensive care, and careful auditing of the quality of outcome. Recently, cogent arguments in favour of redistributing resources towards treatment of these tiny individuals have been advanced on the basis of favourable results from cost–benefit analyses.[1] There is, however, a counter-argument that suggests that there must be some selectivity in applying modern, invasive intensive care techniques. Otherwise, more and more babies will survive, only to be condemned to a poor quality of life.[2] The dilemma is to define where the limits are drawn and by whom. Very immature babies, those with severe congenital abnormalities, and those damaged during pregnancy, delivery, or early post-natal life give rise to most discussion and debate.[3] Neither the weight nor gestational age of babies are precise enough measurements to act as cut-off limits for decision-making.[1] As long ago as the 1930s, a baby weighing 283 g survived. Nowadays, up to 75 per cent of babies in the 700–799 g weight range and up to 40 per cent of those in the 500–599 g category survive. Up to 30 per cent of babies categorized by *obstetric* assessments as gestational age 22 weeks may survive, although no babies categorized as less than 24 weeks' gestation by *neonatal examination* survive. This latter method of assessment has an error of ± 2 weeks and thus the obstetric age assessment is probably as good a guide as any.

The quality of outcome seems to be improving with time although a problem with all longitudinal studies is that they are following a group of children who were given neonatal care that would now be regarded as obsolete. The trend seems to be towards an increase in the absolute numbers of extremely low birthweight survivors with a concomitant increase in the absolute number with disabilities such as cerebral palsy or blindness. However, the proportion of survivors with disabilities is falling and thus the proportion of neurologically normal survivors is increasing. The currently available information supports the idea that babies of birthweight 500 g or more, and 24 weeks gestation or more, should be offered full intensive care support. Those *near* to these weight and age categories who are in a satisfactory condition at birth should also receive full support. Recent changes to legislation in the UK concerned with still birth registration,[4] *in vitro* fertilization,[5] and abortion[6] support this approach. These new laws now use the 24-week gestational age limit in their defining clauses in place of the previously accepted 28-week limit.

The cost–benefit figures for neonatal intensive care are remarkably favourable compared with many other medical therapies.[1] For the baby with congenital anomalies or who has been damaged *in utero* or perinatally, the severity of brain damage is often the main determinant in the decision to embark on intensive care management. The medical staff should take a lead in decision-making and should not leave it up to the parents to decide on their own. At a time of great distress, this is too much of a burden and often, from the parents perspective, a clear view of what is in the best interests of the child will be obscured by the emotional trauma of the situation. Such decisions are best made jointly by medical staff and parents on an individual case-by-case basis. Ethics committees can provide useful guidance and a framework of advice but the decision-making process should not be passed over to them. Parental pressure in favour of futile treatment or non-treatment should be resisted until an agreement is achieved between medical staff and parents which is in the best interests of the child and which is acceptable medically, socially, and legally. Involvement of the courts should be reserved for the difficult cases where serious disagreements occur.

Withdrawal of intensive care treatment that has already begun is sometimes differentiated from witholding intensive care.[3] There is an argument for giving them equal moral standing,[2] in that to withhold treatment when it will not benefit the patient is equivalent to withdrawing it. Conversely, not to start treatment when it is indicated is as wrong as withdrawing it when it is beneficial. In other words, beneficial treatment should be started and not withdrawn, whereas non-beneficial treatment should not be started but *may* be withdrawn. This latter situation often occurs in clinical practice and time must be allowed for staff and relatives to adjust to the inevitable. This subject is considered in more detail in Chapter 4.

Resuscitation should be instituted at birth in all infants of whatever birthweight, maturity, or apparent abnormality to allow time for a considered judgement of the situation by senior personnel. Particularly difficult clinical situations arise when severely asphyxiated infants, very premature babies, or the birth of a living fetus from an elective termination of pregnancy occur. This latter group, if vigorous and spontaneously breathing (which is unlikely, but possible), should be resuscitated and offered intensive care.

Resuscitation in the neonatal intensive care unit (ICU) is usual unless it has been decided that further treatment is futile. Such decisions should be made by senior staff after full consultation with the parents. All involved with the immediate care of the child should be fully informed of the decision.

Where full intensive care support is withdrawn or withheld, the comfort of the child should be the first priority in the care given. Warmth, cleanliness, hygiene, oral feeds or fluids, human touch, and pain relief are all essential components of comfort. In some infants, the process of dying may be prolonged but the quality of the process will be enhanced and time allowed for adaptation by the parents. In certain cases, this process can be accomplished by allowing the family to take the baby home.

Other dilemmas in neonatology occur when medical accidents occur or when deterioration in the infant's condition occurs due to progression of their disease or development of a complication of treatment. A clear, truthful explanation in plain language that the parents can understand is warranted. Clear and witnessed documentation of the incident and the discussion with parents is essential.

2. Resource allocation

Resource limitation is a problem faced by all health care systems with considerable variations in the threshold of provision. An example would be to consider the situation where the neonatal ICU is full and a further admission of a baby who would benefit from intensive care is imminent. Can a rational and ethically sound decision be made about whether this baby should receive intensive care when this will require the withdrawal of support from another baby who is less likely to benefit? Costs and benefits to individual patients, families, and society in general must be weighed but not solely using financial parameters. Centralization of intensive care expertise in large tertiary referral centres leads to improved outcome for the sickest infants and is cheaper and more cost-effective than trying to duplicate such facilities on multiple sites. In an overall debate about intensive care resource allocation, this is a powerful argument. Performance of neonatal and paediatric ICUs needs to be audited using tools which allow comparisons of care for equally sick infants. The decision to divert funding to the best units however requires much more detailed information that is seldom available at present.

3. Consent to treatment

The law gives parents authority to make decisions on behalf of the child provided this proxy consent is exercised reasonably and in the best interests of the infant. In neonatal and paediatric intensive care it is good clinical practice to keep parents and relatives fully informed about the condition of their child, the level of life support, and invasive interventions required. As part of this dialogue, the risks of intensive care interventions should be raised. The level of detail on the 'downside' of intensive care has to be balanced against the distress of the relatives. Certain invasive procedures are regarded as routine by paediatric intensivists (e.g. intubation, ventilation, and insertion of arterial and venous monitoring lines). As technology advances, many would argue that new modes of ventilation, extracorporeal life-support techniques, and new drugs, such as nitric oxide and surfactant, should be regarded as routine. Specific verbal or written consent is often sought for use of these therapies, however, because the risk–benefit ratio is still being evaluated. Specific written consent is sought when a new technique is part of a clinical trial. This can lead to problems if 'control' patients are offered conventional therapy, whereas 'study' patients are offered the new treatment. The ethical window for conducting such studies is only open for a short time after which the new treatment becomes incorporated into the conventional armamentarium, sometimes on fairly anecdotal grounds.

A good example of this phenomenon is the way in which extracorporeal life support has been promoted, with the result that few, if any, sound prospective randomized trials have been conducted to prove benefit over conventional therapy. For life-saving treatments like this, some argue that it is unethical not to offer the treatment. However, agents such as steroids and monoclonal antibody therapy, which were used to treat septic shock on fairly thin scientific but strong anecdotal grounds, are no longer used because prospective randomized controlled trials showed no overall benefit and revealed considerable added risks. It is more ethically acceptable to undertake and invest in well-conducted studies at the outset of a new treatment. Hospital ethics committees have a role to play in only passing properly designed trials. An example of good evaluative work is the introduction of surfactant therapy in neonatal intensive care, although studies are ongoing to clarify the optimum dose and formulation, and which patient subgroups gain most benefit.

In some situations, such as elective admission to intensive care of an older child who is adjudged to be able to understand fully the nature and consequences of the proposed interventions in the ICU, consent may also be sought from the child but the parent or guardian will usually also have to be a party to the discussion. In this type of case, the intensive care management is often a part of the overall surgical management of the child (e.g. repair of congenital heart defect or correction of scoliosis).[7] When children lack the requisite competence to consent as adjudged by the doctor (a result of the judgment in the Gillick case[8]), consent by a person with parental responsibility permits treatment to take place. This responsibility can rest with either parent if they are married to each other, with the mother alone if unmarried, with the natural father if a formal agreement has been reached with the mother or a court has ordered such an arrangement, or with others by court order, care order or emergency protection order.[7]

A child's or parent's refusal of an intensive care intervention are not subject to the same requirements as those for consent.[7,9–11] Society assumes that treatment is proposed because it will bring benefit to the patient. To refuse treatment, the individual must demonstrate understanding 'commensurate with the gravity of the decision . . . The more serious the decision, the greater the capacity required'.[10] Some would say that a child who refuses a life-saving treatment cannot be mature enough to fully understand the implications of their refusal. The courts have the responsibility to act in the child's best interests and will intervene if refusal is unreasonable.[9] Do parents have the right to consent to a critical care treatment against the express wishes of their child? This situation certainly occurs although the scenario has not been tested in court.

Often, life-saving measures have to be commenced in paediatric and neonatal intensive care when the parents are not immediately present. An example would be siting of a chest drain for relief of a tension pneumothorax in a ventilated child. The intervention is a necessity and it will be assumed that any reasonable parent would have given their consent. Frequently, a telephone contact can be made virtually simultaneously by another member of staff but sometimes parents are out of contact. A good unit will forewarn parents of the possibility of rapid changes in their child's clinical condition and the need for minimal delay with interventions. Where it is not possible to gain consent, a note to that effect with reasons for the urgency of the intervention should be made in the case record and a confirmatory note by a second doctor would be advisable. For non-life-saving measures, the intervention may have to be postponed until parental contact can be made.

Refusal by a parent of intensive care treatment or of an intervention may be problematic. Parental refusal of life-saving treatment should be overruled by the child's right to live, but only in an emergency situation. Otherwise, the courts will have to decide.

4. Diagnosis of brain death, and organ donation

The criteria for establishing brainstem death are in principle the same in children over 2 months of age as in adults.[12] Preconditions for applying the tests of brainstem death must be satisfied. After a period of observation in a patient who is comatose and mechanically ventilated for apnoea and in whom the diagnosis of structural brain damage has been established or in whom the immediate cause of coma is known, tests of brainstem function may be performed provided hypothermia, neuromuscular block-ade, drug-induced coma, endocrine, and metabolic disturbances have been excluded. Concomitant measurement of blood levels of barbiturates and other sedative drugs to confirm they are not contributing to coma is useful and full reversal of neuromuscular blocking agents should be confirmed using a nerve stimulator.

Senior staff should undertake the tests on two separate occasions and one should not be primarily involved in the child's care. The pupillary response to light, corneal reflex, vestibulo-ocular reflex, doll's eye reflex, motor response to pain in the distribution of the fifth cranial nerve, gag reflex in response to suctioning, and apnoea in the presence of a normal arterial oxygen level and high arterial carbon dioxide levels ($Pa_{CO_2} > 50$ mmHg; > 7 kPa) are all checked.[12]

For infants less than 2 months of age, it is rarely possible to diag-nose brainstem death and for small babies less than 37 weeks of ges-tational age, the concept of brainstem death is probably inappropriate. Electrophysiological measurements are not often of help given the vagaries of interpretation.

Clearly, the diagnosis of brainstem death must be made before the patient can be considered as an organ donor and thus organ retrieval from children less than 2 months old is unlikely to be achievable. Harvesting of organs from anencephalic donors is also not regarded as being acceptable in most countries, because of the difficulty in defining brainstem death in these infants.

What about donation of healthy organs when the donor is a child? The decision making here is based on an analysis of risks and benefits.[13] The risks involved in donating blood are clearly less than in donating bone marrow, skin, a lobe of liver, or a kidney. This list also follows a scale of regenerative capacity which is a major factor in the risk assessment. These procedures are non-therapeutic as far as the donor is concerned. They are potentially harmful to the donor but also potentially beneficial to the recipient. However, the consideration that the donor may suffer some psychological harm if the donation does not proceed has also been taken into account in previous cases. The donor's level of understanding and the ability to consent must also be considered. In some countries, the courts have looked favourably on cases of organ donation of non-regenerative organs from minors but in the UK and Canada, this is not regarded as being ethically acceptable.[13] Where regenerative tissues are concerned, informed parental consent and the consent of the child donor, if possible, should be obtained. At present, the question of organ donation from child to parent is not regarded as being acceptable but in America, partial liver transplants between parent and child have been carried out, a procedure with considerable potential risks for both.

5. Research

Most children in intensive care units are unable to give consent to research, and consent must be sought from a parent or legal guardian. However, some older children who are to be admitted to intensive care electively, for example after scoliosis surgery, may well be able to give consent to research. Guidelines, such as those published by the British Paediatric Association[14] provide a sound foundation. They recognize the distinction between therapeutic research (where direct benefit may accrue to the patient) and non-therapeutic research (where no such benefit will occur but where benefit to future patients may). The benefits to these or future patients must be balanced against the risks involved in the research.[15] Thus, research should be divided into minimal-, low- or, high-risk categories. Much useful minimal-risk research can be carried out in neonatal and paediatric intensive care by careful observation, collection of physiological data, or sampling of blood or urine from indwelling monitoring lines or catheters. Limits should be placed on the volume of blood sampled for the purposes of research as iatrogenic anaemia due to sampling does occur in smaller children and in those who are in intensive care for long periods. A limit of 1 ml/kg (10 ml, maximum) is workable for most research but could be relaxed for those children undergoing extracorporeal life support. Minimal-risk research is usually justifiable for therapeutic and non-therapeutic projects. Low-risk procedures which cause brief pain or discomfort may be justifiable for research purposes alone but in intensive care situations it should be possible to provide adequate analgesia and sedation for these interventions. Some thought must be given to alternative ways of gaining the same information which do not involve an extra needle stick or injection. Indwelling monitoring lines circumvent many of these problems. Topical local anaesthetic cream should be used to prepare the skin in advance of venepunctures or lumbar punctures for research. High-risk procedures should only be carried out for diagnostic or therapeutic reasons with the aim of benefiting that child. There are potential grey areas between low-and high-risk categories which must be considered. An example would be an investigation of a new drug in the paediatric or neonatal intensive care population. Often, the risks of administering the drug are not quantifiable and extrapolations from adult practice are not always valid. It may be justifiable in the context of a life-saving situation to try the new drug as a 'last resort' measure for that particular named patient. Usually no special licence is required but informed parental consent must be obtained and documented. Ethics committee review of trials and adherence to the advice from drug regulatory authorities regarding clinical trial certification will be required for studies in neonatal and paediatric intensive care.[16] Pharmaceutical companies are reluctant to support trials in these clinical areas because of worries about costly product liability claims. However, critically ill children are at risk of becoming 'therapeutic orphans'[17] and losing out on potentially beneficial treatments unless clinicians and licensing authorities insist on properly conducted trials. The doctor has a duty to act in the best interests of the child and not to cause harm. Fully informed consent from the parent or guardian (and child if possible) is required and must be on the basis of as detailed an assessment of risks and benefits as is possible. Parents must not be pressurized by only offering appropriate treatment to their child if they agree to participation in the study. A new treatment may, however, only be available as part of a trial and this must not be construed as putting pressure on the parents to consent.

For non-therapeutic research in children there are no firm legal rules or precedents and ethical principles determine practice. Some hold that minimal-risk non-therapeutic research is permissible if the child is over 7 years old and gives consent. Others hold that only therapeutic research should be allowed as any medical procedure carries a risk of harm and the overriding consideration is the child's welfare. A possible justification for non-therapeutic research is that the difference in physiology between neonates, children, and adults requires separate study. Society as a whole or that child himself in later life may benefit from the knowledge gained by the research. However, the interests of science and society should not take precedence over the well-being of the individual.[10] Is there a level of negligible risk that would produce huge societal benefits? Can a reasonable parent give consent in these circumstances? If the child himself or herself understands the risk–benefit ratio and the implications for him or herself and society, should he or she be allowed to agree to non-therapeutic research? This *may* be acceptable if the risk is very small but is less likely to be acceptable as the degree of risk rises. The problem is where to set the limits. For the neonatal and paediatric intensive care population, the local ethics committee has a particularly important role in striking a balance. Often, the practical problem is that the degree of additional risk due to the research is difficult to judge in this inherently risky environment and in this particularly ill group of children. It is vital that research workers honestly reveal potential risks for a reasonable individual to consider before being asked to give consent. Legally valid consent is both freely given and informed. No financial inducements or emotional pressure should be applied and time must be allowed for families to consider and discuss among themselves whether they should consent or not. They must be free to change their mind without penalty and without giving a reason. They must also be assured that their child's treatment will not be prejudiced by their decision to withdraw from the research.[14] Parental involvement in the research and common sense explanations as the research proceeds are vital, particularly during longer or more difficult studies. Leaflets or handouts for parents are helpful in keeping the parent fully informed and must be produced in plain language with a minimum of technical terms. These documents should be scrutinized and approved by the ethics committee. It is also beneficial to relay the results of the research to the family in plain language so that they get a sense of what has been achieved.

A good test is always to ask: 'If this was my child, would *I* give *my* consent?'

These legal and ethical issues have an impact daily in neonatal and paediatric intensive care practice. The underlying principle is to act at all times in the best interests of the child within locally determined medical, social, and legal mores.

Notes

1. Roberton, N.R.C. (1993). Should we look after babies less than 800 g? *Archives of Disease in Childhood*, **68**, 326–9.
2. Campbell, A.G.M. (1994) Ethical problems in neonatal care. In *Textbook of neonatology*, (ed. N.R.C. Roberton), pp. 43–8. Churchill-Livingstone, Edinburgh.
3. Doyal, L., and Wilsher, D. (1991). Towards guidelines for witholding and withdrawal of life prolonging treatment in neonatal medicine. *Archives of Disease in Childhood*, **70**, F66–F70.
4. Forrest, GC. (1994) Perinatal death. In *Textbook of neonatology*, (ed. N.R.C. Roberton), pp. 75–80. Churchill-Livingstone, Edinburgh.
5. BMA (British Medical Association) (1993). Reproduction and genetic technology. In *Medical ethics today*, pp. 97–131. BMJ Publishing Group, London.
6. BMA (British Medical Association) (1993). Reproduction and genetic technology. In *Medical ethics today*, p. 106. BMJ Publishing Group, London.
7. BMA (British Medical Association) (1993). Children and young people. In *Medical ethics today*, pp. 69–96. BMJ Publishing Group, London.
8. *Gillick* v. *Norfolk and Wisbech Area Health Authority* [1985] 3 WLR 830, All ER 402.
9. Pace, NA. (1991). Legal and ethical considerations of consent in children: implications for anaesthetists. *Paediatric Anaesthesia*, **1**, 21–4.
10. BMA (British Medical Association) (1993). Consent and refusal. In *Medical ethics today*, pp. 23–24. BMJ Publishing Group, London.
11. Per Lord Donaldson in *Re T* [1992] 4 All ER 649.
12. British Paediatric Association (1990) *Working party report on the diagnosis of brainstem death in children*. British Paediatric Association, London.
13. Pace, N.A. (1992). Legal and ethical considerations of organ donation in children: implications for anaesthetists. *Paediatric Anaesthesia*, **2**, 231–3.
14. British Paediatric Association. (1992) *Guidelines for the ethical conduct of medical research involving children*. British Paediatric Association, London.
15. Pace, N.A. (1992). Legal and ethical considerations of research in children: implications for anaesthetists. *Paediatric Anaesthesia*, **2**, 17–21.
16. Department of Health and Social Security (1968). *Medicines Act 1968. A guide to the provisions affecting doctors and dentists*. HMSO, London.
17. Kauffman, R.E. (1991). Fentanyl, fads, and folly: who will adopt the therapeutic orphans? *Journal of Pediatrics*, **119**, 588–9.

9

The Nursing Perspective

Kath M. Melia

Ethical issues that arise for nurses working in intensive care are, it could be argued, in some ways different from ethical issues in nursing in general in that they have a particular focus dictated by the setting. The work of intensive care, by definition, suggests that patients are likely to be vulnerable, possibly not conscious, and highly unlikely to be able to conduct their lives for the time being in the autonomous fashion to which they are accustomed. To be in need of intensive care is to have suspended life's general order and to subject oneself to the care of others. As the professional group taking over the care and the day-to-day decisions about how life will be lived, the challenge presented to nurses by the intensive care patient carries many of the hallmarks of any nursing challenge, the main one being to do for patients that which they would do for themselves were they able (Henderson 1966).[1] It is, therefore, the thesis of this chapter that the ethical considerations for nursing practice in an intensive care unit (ICU) will not be very different from those arising elsewhere. In other words, the ethical dimension of nursing care is sufficiently fundamental that it will override any preoccupations driven by the setting.

It might be useful, then, to look at the ethical dimension of nursing work and the principles that underpin nursing practice before going on to examine the aspects of intensive care, which might lead us to have to question the argument that nursing ethics in intensive care are the same as nursing ethics elsewhere. There is a tendency to suppose that if an area exists where there is a concentration of ethical issues the ICU will be that area. Whether we want to think about nursing, medical, or health care ethics, the ICU is likely to come to mind as the obvious hotbed for ethical debate. It was in these areas of high technology that some of the early questions which brought ethics into the forefront of medicine arose. The arrival of life-support machines and development of transplantation techniques led to the need for definitions of brain death. The possibility of transplanting ever more complex organs gives rise to ethical issues surrounding the care of the donor and the family. In other words, the issues surrounding new technologies go beyond potential risks and the ethicality of the transplant, or whatever, itself. All of these developments took place in the ICU and so it is not surprising that it is these units from which the debates are thought to stem, indeed they are often the source of the debate. It is also true to say that questions of cost and resource allocation arise in the ICU. Questions of costs and debates about allocation of resources arise all over the health care service, but the intensive care areas are commonly thought to be the most expensive and possibly offering the least value for money on any utilitarian analysis. However, it is equally true to say that other areas of practice tend to make comparisons with the cost of intensive care and so the ethics of resource allocation is a health service-wide debate in which intensive care serves as a rather prominent bench-mark.

We should not let the setting of high technology and advanced medical practice lead us away from the basis of ethics in health care. It is possible to find foundations and principles that can give us some insights into what the moral issues are and how we can look to these in order to guide practice in intensive care in much the same way that we might look to these principles in other less dramatic areas of practice. There is a considerable literature on nursing ethics which seeks to lay out the principles on which nursing practice can be based. The nursing ethics literature is not concerned to tell nurses how to behave, rather it is concerned with opening up the issues and employing the language of moral philosophy in order to make ethical debate possible. If nurses are to be able to discuss the rights and wrongs of their practice in settings where they are not in ultimate control and where their personal values may be in conflict with those of colleagues and patients, it is essential that a common means of debate and discussion be found. Moral philosophy provides just that formulation. Campbell (1984, p. 9)[2] in recommending ethical theory to practitioners in health care says:

All ethical theories return at one point or another to particular situations in order to exemplify the concepts being discussed or to discover the practical implications of a principle being formulated. It is the movement back and forth between the particular and the general which gives the subject a potential value for the contemporary dilemmas of those working in medicine.

It is generally true to say that any debate or discussion of nursing ethics which starts with a particular case will sooner or later come around to a discussion of the principles on which the issue rests. These principles are in most discussions: *Justice, beneficence* (duty to care), and *autonomy* (respect for persons).

1. Justice

This principle concerns equitable allocation of resources and nursing time and effort relative to objectively observed need. Justice is clearly a lot more complicated than that, but as a basis for discussion of a fair use of nursing skills, it is an appropriate starting point.

2. Beneficence

Beneficence, or a duty to care, is a principle that underpins nursing care, one which Florence Nightingale espoused when she exhorted nurses first to do the sick no harm. A duty to care is perhaps more problematic, when we try to determine when care is appropriate. The vexed questions around euthanasia and the proper course of action in persistent vegetative state (PVS) lead us to wonder when to care is indeed to do one's duty. When patients request action which the medical and nursing professions feel that they cannot offer it is hard to see whether patients interests are being served. Gillett (1993, p. 263)[3] describes very forcefully this notion of uncertainty combined with the need to take a decision about action, or indeed non-action, when in, discussing the need for sensitivity to patients' real wishes, he says:

we do not want a 'heal with steel' or 'give me the serum rhubarb!' mentality to hijack our practice in the area of terminal care. Medicine at this juncture must have a clear view of its own limitations, it has no answers, it can palliate and to some extent offer release but the tragedy of human death, even when the time seems right, precludes any talk of success.

Nursing has a problem here too, for although it is indeed medicine that requires the clear view because medicine is ultimately responsible for decisions about care, nurses are very much involved in that care. It is the nursing staff that are most of the time with the patients—they are involved in decisions to which they may have been party, however, they have no legal right to make a decision. This is a position that nurses do not always accept and sometimes engage in ethical debate which is really something of an attack on medical practice and has more to do with power disputes between the professions than anything else.

3. Autonomy

The third principle at the base of nursing practice is autonomy (respect for persons). This includes confidentiality and has to do with having respect for a person's right to autonomy. This principle does not give rise to objections as it would be difficult to make a case that argued against respecting persons. However, it does pose difficulties in terms of practice when patients cannot express themselves. Nurses often have to act in ways which they judge to be in a patient's best interest; it is difficult to do this if there is no way of knowing what a patient would consider to be the best course of action. As in many areas of care, this problem is eased slightly when the patient has known the nurses for some time, for instance, in terminal care. However, if it is an emergency situation that brings a patient into the ICU the staff really are working in the dark. There is both comfort and unease to be derived from the fact that we may never know if we acted in the 'right' way for some patients.

4. Nursing in the ICU

The existence of these principles just discussed does not mean that nursing practice can proceed untroubled as they only provide guidelines. Action requires reflection. It is also apparent reading the principles that there is potential for conflict between them. A duty of care, for example, may well lead a professional to act in a way which would not be in keeping with respect for persons. One might, however, as the pro-euthanasia movement does, argue that the ultimate right to determine how a life is lived rests with the patient. Nurses and doctors alike then have to look hard at the question of what their practice entails—the rights of one group do not automatically bring with them duties for another group. In other words, a right to die claimed by a section of society does not bring with it a duty on the part of health care professionals to help secure that death.

Thus far, we have not mentioned the ICU specifically in relation to these basic principles on which medical and nursing ethics rests. Before moving on to raise some questions that may make the case for special ICU nursing ethics we should emphasize the place of power in the debate. Whenever multidisciplinary decisions take place, there is more than a difference of perspective at stake. It can be argued that the ethical issues that arise from clinical situations are the same for medicine and nursing but that the differences which give rise to discussion have to do with responses to the situation. For example, the decision to discontinue treatment or to withdraw life support will rest on the same kinds of debates for nurses and doctors. Once the decision has been taken there will continue to be the same concerns expressed by both professional groups. However, the nurses experience a more continuous kind of contact with the patient than in general do the doctors, although in the ICU this argument is less forceful than it might be in other areas of care. On the other hand, it is the doctors who carry the responsibility, importantly the legal responsibility, for the treatment and outcome, whereas the nurses may have expressed opinions about the nature of that treatment. Issues of power clearly arise because although we have come a long way from the handmaiden-to-medicine approach, and team decisions are now commonplace in the ICU, it is none the less true to say that the medical members of the team carry the legal responsibility for the diagnostic and treatment decisions. This clear-cut legal position on responsibility for patients is rather more problematic in practice, for both doctors and other health care professionals, notably and of interest in this context, for nurses.

There is a variety of experience which ensues once ethical decisions have been taken and it is on these considerations that we usually focus when the case is made for having nursing ethics as a separate entity from medical ethics. I have argued elsewhere (Melia 1994)[4] that this case is more apparent than real and that in the age of multidisciplinary care we should be looking to co-operation in all areas including that of ethics. A notion of health care ethics with a focus on the patient and society rather than the professions would be a useful goal. Intensive care, with its emphasis on teamwork is an ideal setting in which to promote health care ethics as a multidisciplinary enterprise rather than as a major arena in which to battle out medical versus nursing ethics.

We have taken as a starting point for this discussion of ethical issues involved in intensive care nursing the position that issues will be, at heart, similar if not identical to those that arise more generally in nursing. That is to say, the central issues range around the question how should nurses caring for patients behave with respect to those patients? In what respect are patients compromised in terms of autonomy and self-determination when they place themselves in the hands of professional carers, in this case in the hands of nurses? Having posed the questions we need to address them in terms of how nurses approach this aspect of their work. What mechanisms are there in professional education and practice that ensure that this dimension of nursing care is addressed? It could be argued that these questions have already been answered in a general sense because nursing practice, when we come to examine its moral base, rests on the three principles namely, *justice, beneficence*, and *respect for persons*.

5. Challenges to nursing ethics

One of the reasons that nursing ethics in an ICU might be thought to be different from nursing ethics in a wider sense is the tendency to consider ethics in terms of dilemmas rather than in terms of less headline-grabbing moral choice. Writers on ethics and moral philosophy, when discussing health care, tend to proceed in terms of a consideration of moral dilemmas. That is to say, situations where whatever course of action is determined on some set of moral principles will be compromised—there is no neat solution, hence the dilemma. Moral choices which we make in every day in practice are, on the other hand, less dramatic. Nevertheless, the moral basis of nursing care rests perhaps more on everyday moral choice than it does on the decisions taken when dilemmas occur. Clearly, there is room for both approaches in ethical debate, dilemmas exist and the academic debates centring on them serve to help us to focus our thoughts.

The issues which raise questions for the premise that intensive care ethics is not really any different from nursing ethics in general are those which arise from the technical possibilities of medical science coupled with a society which has a problem with its mortality. We might consider some of the particular circumstances which could call for a different nursing ethics, for example, '*heroic*' life-saving measures and the *prolongation of life*, including the particularly difficult cases of PVS.

Questions of *heroic measures* are complicated by the fact that the person is frequently incapable of expressing a view. It is difficult for nurses to act in such a way as to respect a person's autonomy and wishes when they are not being expressed. Advance directives offer some help, but these are far from universal and do not render a situation problem-free. The ICU is most likely to be dealing with the next of kin. This in itself brings problems. The next of kin is often treated as if there were some legal status attached to the person who is regarded in a day-to-day sense by the nursing staff as the patient's outside contact. Also, in practice, the next of kin is the first person to be consulted if decisions are to be made or information imparted. Where a patient is seriously ill and possibly incapable of taking decisions this person is all the more important. The reliance on the next of kin as the patient's proxy is an interesting feature of a health care system which strives to make patient autonomy and confidentiality paramount (Melia 1987).[5]

Nurses in intensive care have particular problems when it comes to prolongation of life. They have to continue with the care of patients who have become, or are well on the way to becoming, what many would regard as non-persons. Any amount of discussion about the sanctity of life and personhood does not, for many people, remove the difficulties involved in caring for patients who in many ways present as no more than bodies. The problem does not go away with the declaration that life is not for us to take. We have to weigh up the alternatives. Are we causing more harm by continuing as if the person is alive, when in fact they cannot enjoy the life that those in the population enjoy? Is it sensible to evaluate a life with reference to what is natural when the life that we are discussing is being maintained by unnatural means? The problem with the notion of 'naturalness' is that it is a relative concept, things that we take for granted today were once considered not to be natural, indeed were not possible.

The case of Anthony Bland led to a wide debate about the withdrawal of nutrition and fluids, which culminated in a House of Lords Select Committee being set up to consider the use of life-sustaining treatments and euthanasia.[6] In the Bland case, the nurses were faced with a particularly long haul of care for a patient whose life was recognized by almost everyone involved, including his parents, to carry no meaning or quality. The law protects life to the extent that doctors in this case, with the consent and support of relatives and the large majority of the nursing staff, had to go to an English court to obtain permission for the withdrawal of nutrition. The Select Committee discussed many issues but failed to come up with a unanimous view on the central question about the withdrawal of nutrition. Having stated that:

we do not therefore distinguish between withholding and withdrawal of treatment, in our discussion of treatment limiting decisions,

the Committee go on to say that:

treatment-limiting decisions in respect of an incompetent patient should be taken jointly by all those involved in his or her care, including the entire health care team and the family or other people closest to the patient. Their guiding principle should be that a treatment may be judged inappropriate if it will add nothing to the patient's well-being as a person.

However, when it came to the issue of defining artificial means of feeding the Committee side-stepped the question saying:

Nor do we think it helpful to attempt a firm distinction between treatment and personal care, implying that the former may be limited and the latter not. The two are part of a continuum, and such boundary as there is between them shifts as practice evolves and particularly as the wider role of nursing develops. This boundary is one which the courts were required to try to define in the case of Tony Bland, and that gave rise to much debate about whether nutrition and hydration, even when given by invasive methods, may ever be regarded as a treatment which in certain circumstances it may be inappropriate to initiate or continue.

In one of the less useful passages in the whole report they say that:

this question has caused us great difficulty, with some members of the Committee taking one view and some another, and we have not been able to reach a conclusion. ... We consider that progressive development and ultimate acceptance of the notion that some treatment is inappropriate should make it unnecessary to consider the withdrawal of nutrition and hydration, except in circumstances where its administration is in itself evidently burdensome to the patient.

This report is of general interest to an ethical debate in health care and to debates on intensive care, in particular. The stress on joint decision-making and consultation would support the idea that nursing ethics should not be regarded as a separate entity from medical ethics. It is also interesting to note that in the area with which the Committee had most difficulty (i.e. the question of definition of artificial feeding), they introduce the developing role of the nurse as part of their argument for not distinguishing between treatment and care. It is not altogether clear what significance they placed on this, only that the 'wider role of the nurse' is mentioned.

Most of these issues, which at first glance seem to have to do with intensive care ethics, are not so different from the issues that arise in other areas. If we keep a close eye on the similarities in the situations that arise in intensive care, compared with those in other areas, and do not let the assumption that intensive care is so very different and dilemma-prone lead us away from the importance of everyday moral choice in intensive care, we can go back to the three basic principles, namely, *justice, beneficence*, and *autonomy* (respect for persons).

6. Conclusion

The dramatic heroic life-saving situations which occur in intensive care lead us back to respect for persons and the conflicts that following this principle lead to. Informed consent is an ever-present issue in such situations. The same principle is of relevance in contemplating questions of PVS. Justice is an all-pervading concept which brings us back to the very basis of nursing ethical debates.

At heart then, all these issues come back to the same principles that nursing in general relies on in order to focus on its moral basis. We do not need to create a special ethics for intensive care, what we work with already in nursing will suffice, it is only the cases and the contexts that differ, the principles transcend the settings. The same point was made by the Select Committee[6] on the question of PVS when they noted that similar issues have been around for a long time in all areas of medicine:

It is already incumbent on doctors and other staff caring for the patient to consider very carefully whether any new treatment they are about to provide for the patient is in his/her best interest. This is an important general principle not confined to patients in persistent vegetative state (PVS) or who may develop PVS.

Finally, it is worthwhile considering a possible consequence of regarding intensive care ethics as a different entity from nursing ethics in general. It could be that a focus on the dramatic and fast moving pace of intensive care may cause us to give undue emphasis to the dilemma aspect of ethical debate and less to the less obvious everyday issues of moral choice. The case of Anthony Bland involves the two aspects, early drama and then a long, slow, and, for the friends and family, painful process through a life-supported limbo to a tragic, but in the final circumstances welcomed death.

The principles of respect for persons and autonomy clearly have relevance throughout the four years of Anthony Bland's care. We need to keep a balance between a consideration of dilemmas and everyday moral choice. In the ICU setting it is important not to let the high-technology context and the sense of imminent dilemma overshadow the consideration of the moral choices which are very much the style of intensive care nursing.

Notes

1. Henderson, V. (1966). *The nature of nursing* Collier Macmillan, London.
2. Campbell, A.V. (1984). *Moral dilemmas in medicine*. Churchill Livingstone, Edinburgh.
3. Gillett, G. (1993). Learning to do no harm. *Journal of Medicine and Philosophy*, 18, 253–68.
4. Melia, K.M. (1994). The task of nursing ethics. *Journal of Medical Ethics*, 20, pp. 7–11.
5. Melia, K.M. (1987). Relatively distant. *Nursing Times*, 83, pp. 26–8.
6. House of Lords (1994). *Report of the Select Committee on Medical Ethics*. Vol. I: Report, Vol. II: Oral evidence. HL Paper 21.1. HMSO, London. (1994). Review. House of Lords on care of the dying. *Bulletin of Medical Ethics*, No. 95, 13–16.

10
Ventilating Patients for Organ Donation

Malcolm G. Booth and Peter G.M. Wallace

1. Introduction

The problems relating to the diagnosis of brain stemdeath and the provision of organ donors have been addressed elsewhere. This chapter discusses the legal and ethical problems relating to a new development in the procurement of human organs for transplantation.

In the UK there has been an effort in recent years to ensure that relatives of all potential donors dying in the intensive care unit (ICU) are approached for permission to harvest organs after death. Despite this there is still a shortage of organs nationally. At the end of 1992 there were 4361 patients awaiting renal transplantation in the UK. This is increasing by almost 10 per cent per annum.[1] Although several different methods of recruiting more donors have been suggested, a new proposal termed 'interventional' or 'elective ventilation', aims to utilize those patients expected to die from massive cerebrovascular accidents who are not usually admitted to the ICU.

Organ retrieval to date has been guided by two moral principles. The first of these is the 'dead donor rule'; which is that vital organs may only be taken from dead patients and that conversely no patient shall be harmed in the procurement of organs. The second guideline has been that the care of the living patient will never be adversely affected by the requirements of potential organ recipients.[2]

Currently, organ donation is from patients admitted to the ICU in their own interests who are subsequently diagnosed brainstem dead prior to the decision as to whether that patient is, or is not, a suitable organ donor. Patients are admitted to the ICU for treatment or diagnosis with no reference or regard to their suitability as future organ donors. Treatment is started in the patient's interest and it is only after irreversible coma is diagnosed progressing to brainstem death that organ donation is considered. The diagnosis of brainstem death is made before the involvement of the transplant team, therefore avoiding any appearance of advance selection of possible donors.

There are, however, many patients admitted to hospital severely ill who are allowed to die peacefully in the ward because admission to the ICU will not alter their outcome. Obviously, many of these, for reasons such as infection, renal or cardiovascular failure, may be unsuitable for use as organ donors. A group of patients, however, who might be 'suitable' for organ donation are those dying of primary irreversible intracranial haemorrhage in whom it has been decided that there will be no benefit from intensive care. As noted, some patients suffering a cerebrovascular accident (CVA) are already admitted to the ICU and ventilated to permit diagnosis. Once the diagnosis of irreversible CVA has been established they will progress to a point where brainstem death can be diagnosed. In the UK, 14.6 per cent of organ donors are patients who have died of CVAs having been admitted to the ICU as part of their management.[3] Patients, however, may have had the same diagnosis made before the need for artificial ventilation arises. Once a diagnosis of massive and irreversible CVA has been made artificial ventilation will not be in the patient's direct interests when respiratory function fails nor will it alter their outcome.

Interventional ventilation involves transferring these patients previously allowed to die in the ward and admits them to the ICU for non-therapeutic ventilation with the sole intent of harvesting their organs after brainstem death occurs and has been diagnosed. This practice raises several issues: namely the question of consent, the fact that interventions are not in the patient's best interests, and the possibility of compromising the patient's expected demise.

2. The Exeter Protocol

There has only been one study of the use of interventional or elective ventilation published to date (Feest *et al.*).[4] The details are described below.

A retrospective study of patients dying of CVA in a district general hospital revealed that in a 12-month period there were 38 deaths in patients aged 70 years or younger. Of these, six had been admitted to the ICU because respiratory arrest had occurred immediately prior to or on admission to hospital before any management decisions had been made. Patients admitted to the ICU were ventilated to allow diagnosis and treatment of unexplained coma. Of the six patients who died in the ICU, five were suitable to be organ donors. In two cases, permission was refused and three went on to become donors. The other 32 died on medical or geriatric wards. Of these 32 ward deaths, 24 would not have been suitable for elective transfer to the ICU in an attempt to harvest organs (because of either sudden unexpected death or a gradual deterioration to death, for example, pneumonia) or were not medically suitable to be donors. The remaining eight patients all died within 36 hours of injury or hospital admission. These eight patients could have been potential donors had they been admitted to the ICU for elective ventilation.

A protocol (Table 10.1) was developed to allow the retrieval of organs from patients not admitted in their own interests to the ICU but who seem likely to die from CVA within 48 hours. The protocol allowed the transfer to the ICU of some of these patients for ventilatory support until brain death occurred, was diagnosed, and thereafter organ harvesting arranged.

Table 10.1 The Exeter Protocol

There is no age limit for organ donation, patients over 70 years old may
be suitable.

Criteria for identification of patients with intracranial vascular accidents as potential
organ donors
- Characteristic mode of onset: sudden with rapid development of coma
- Progressive decline in conscious level
- Deep coma: lack of withdrawal response to painful stimuli
- Intravascular accident confirmed by computed tomography desirable

Exclusion: reversible causes of coma

Procedure: this sequence of events must be strictly observed
- Junior medical staff discuss case with consultant concerned
- Consultant or nominee discuss suitability of patient with member of
  transplant team
- If patient suitable, discuss with consultant in charge of the ICU
- If all are agreed, consultant physician or nominee should approach relatives

Approach to relatives: this must include discussion of:
- Physician's belief that patient is unlikely to recover
- Request for organ donation
- Transfer to the ICU as appropriate for management of organ donation
- Possibility of patient leaving the ICU for the ward if he/she ceases to be
  suitable donor

Management in the ICU
- Degree of intensive treatment is for discussion between consultant physician
  and consultant in the ICU

The protocol was described as follows. If a patient was admitted to a medical
or geriatric ward diagnosed as having suffered a CVA such that survival for
more than 48 hours was unlikely and no therapy was possible then he or she
could be entered into the protocol. Reversible causes of coma were excluded
and the diagnosis confirmed by computed tomography (CT) scan if possible.
The consultant physician in charge thereafter discussed the case with a member
of the transplant team as to the suitability of the patient as a donor. If this was
agreed then the ICU consultant would be approached about the availability of

a bed in the ICU. At this point the relatives would be told about the expected death of the patient and a request for organ donation made. The relatives would also be told that if for any reason the patient became unsuitable as a donor then he would transferred out of the ICU and back to the original ward. Permission granted, the patient would be transferred to the ICU, ventilated when required, brain death confirmed, and organ retrieval organized.

During the first 19 months of the protocol 11 patients were notified as possible donors. Nine patients were transferred to the ICU and eight became organ donors. The ninth patient was never ventilated, being discharged from the ICU after five days and died the next day. There were two refusals for transfer to the ICU. Of the 9 patients admitted to ICU under the protocol, four cases did not follow the strict guidelines laid down. This was because the patients' condition declined rapidly before the recommended sequence of steps had been completed and the expected death would have intervened if ventilation had not been commenced. In one case, the relatives suggested organ donation before it was known if the patient was suitable. Discussion with the consultant was not possible in one instance, and in 2 patients, the relatives were not available to grant permission. In the 19-month period, the protocol resulted in the retrieval of 16 kidneys, two livers, one heart, and two sets of heart valves. The authors maintain that this represents, on a national scale, 33.4 kidneys per million population per year as compared with the present UK transplant rate of 19.8 per million.

Although the Exeter Protocol offers a possible solution to the dilemma of organ procurement it poses many ethical and legal questions. We wish to discuss the argument both for and against interventional ventilation.

Following the publication of Feest *et al.*'s paper in the *Lancet*[4] there was considerable reaction in the medical press both for and against the idea. Committees of the British Medical Association and the British Transplant Society considered the issues involved. Both reported in favour of elective ventilation of certain dying patient to obtain organs under strict guidelines, as did the Royal College of Physicians of London.[5]

3. The case for interventional ventilation

The case in favour of elective ventilation is simple and emotive. Surveys suggest that over 70 per cent of the public would like their organs to be used after death.[6] Normally, only those dying on a ventilator in the ICU can do so. The majority of these are identified, although 6 per cent of patients are overlooked as potential donors.[7] Approximately 30 per cent of families approached refuse donation. A reduction in this refusal rate is probably possible but even an opt-out system would not produce sufficient organs to fulfil current requirements.[7–10] Interventional ventilation by electively ventilating suitable dying patients prior to death, when it would not be contemplated as part of their treatment, may ensure more patients become donors once brainstem death is confirmed. The supply of kidneys could increase by over 50 per cent if the experience in Exeter is repeated nationally. This would meet the demand for renal transplantation.

Many of the deaths in the ICU are of a relatively young population who should have had many productive years ahead of them. To relatives, the person's death is unjustifiable and totally pointless. Organ donation, however, gives some purpose to the loss and so helps relatives cope with grief. This will also apply to the relatives of donors resulting from interventional ventilation who are, from the Exeter experience, on average older than those diagnosed brainstem dead following trauma.[11]

Many would say that if society is in a position to offer a cure for a major disease process then it is morally bound to do so.[12] Patients being proposed as potential candidates for elective ventilation are those diagnosed as suffering from a fatal and irreversible disease process. They will die come what may. It is argued that even if patients are beyond any medical help, as a member of society, it is in their interest, and certainly in the continuing society's interest, that their organs be retrieved. Although they will not benefit directly, the welfare of other individuals and society will be enhanced.

The principle of putting society's needs first contradicts the principle of respecting an individual's right of autonomy. There are, however, examples of the common good taking precedence, such as the immunization against rubella for girls, although it is not a principle usually applied in medicine. The Declaration of Geneva of the World Medical Association binds the physician with words: 'The health of my patient will be my first consideration', and the International code of Medical Ethics claims: 'A physician shall act only in the patient's interest'.[13] Also, the Declaration of Helsinki states, 'biomedical research involving human subjects should be preceded by careful assessment of predictable risks in comparison with foreseeable benefits to the subject or to others. Concern for the interests of the subject must always prevail over the interest of science and society'.[13]

One relevant medical example of putting society first is clinical research in the ICU. Research continues in all branches of medicine to improve treatment and evaluate new forms of therapy. All patients included in a research project must be informed of the aims, methods, anticipated benefits, and potential hazards of the study. No form of coercion must be used to recruit volunteers either financial or special treatment. Volunteers must sign a consent form for the study and be able to withdraw at any time without that affecting the standard of their treatment.

Clinical research in the ICU is no different; but who consents to the patient's inclusion? Not the individual in the majority of instances. Despite this, however, a lot of clinical research involving ICU patients is being carried out. The usual method of obtaining 'consent' is to approach the family, discuss the planned investigation emphasizing that it should do no harm, and although the patient may derive no benefit the interests of future patients might be helped.

In the case of interventional ventilation the British Medical Association publication on medical ethics states that, 'respect for individual's autonomy could be compromised by instituting procedures not to benefit the donor but to maintain organ quality, and that this must be weighed against the potential for benefiting many organ recipients and saving lives'.[14] This does seem to condone putting society's interests ahead of the individual's in certain circumstances and contradicts statements from other institutions, although it seems to suggest a degree of uncertainty.

The case in favour of the elective ventilation of dying patients in order to obtain their organs for transplantation may be summarized as follows. It will provide organs needed to treat chronic irreversible organ failure, whilst providing grieving relatives with purpose to the unexpected death of a loved one. Those contributing have, by definition, no further interest in life but may benefit in general by parts of their body offering others a future. It will allow patients and doctors to meet their responsibilities to society as a whole, including patients waiting for organ transplantation. Although stressful and requiring some organization each interventional ventilation patient could benefit five recipients which represents a very high reward.

4. The case against interventional ventilation

There are two accepted definitions of death in the UK. These are the traditional clinical one of cessation of respiratory and cardiac function, and brainstem death based on demonstrating the loss of brainstem reflexes.

The diagnosis of brainstem death, since its introduction in 1979, has been accepted by most of the medical fraternity.[15] This equates brainstem death with clinical death and allows cessation of artificial life support.[16] There appears to be some confusion among the public as to when death actually occurs. An example of this was the reporting of the death of Tim Parry, a schoolboy injured in the Warrington bombing in the spring of 1993. When he was pronounced brainstem-dead and the life support switched off, it was reported in the media that his family stayed with him whilst he 'died'. This suggests that he died after life support was withdrawn. The time of death in these cases is, in fact, when the second brain-death test is carried out.

Even doctors involved in transplantation may misunderstand the time of death. Regarding the onset of apnoea as the time of death is such a misunderstanding. Thus, Nicholls and Riad wrote, in defence of interventional ventilation, that 'such patients die when breathing ceases; elective ventilation does not prolong the act of dying, for one is ventilating a corpse'.[17] This a fundamental misinterpretation.

Death occurs on the cessation of respiratory *and* cardiac activity or may be diagnosed by brainstem testing. If artificial ventilation is not instituted the apnoeic patient will die naturally of cardiac arrest secondary to hypoxia.

Commencing ventilation maintains oxygenation and cardiac function. If ventilation is continued death may only then be presumed following brainstem death testing. Clearly, interventional ventilation prolongs the natural process of dying in these patients by delaying the diagnosis of death until brainstem death can be confirmed

There is a fundamental difference with interventional ventilation compared to traditional organ donation. With traditional practice, it is clearly understood that acceptance for organ donation occurs after death and that primary intervention was for that patient's benefit. This is not the case with interventional ventilation.

5. Consent and the patient's best interests

One persuasive argument against interventional ventilation is the problem of obtaining legal consent. In adults, the only person able to give, or withhold, consent for any medical intervention is the individual concerned. As already stated, patients likely to be recruited for interventional ventilation are admitted to hospital unconscious.

It is normal practice, when treating an unconscious patient, to discuss the treatment options available with the close family. Planned procedures are explained and the relatives are often asked to sign a consent form on behalf of the patient. Although this is courteous, there is no provision under law for one adult to give consent for medical treatment on behalf of another adult,[18] (Medical and Dental Defence Union of Scotland, personal communication). However, speaking to relatives may provide information about the patient's own attitude(s) concerning treatment and also helps to establish that the doctor's attitude and actions will be reasonable (this is important should a decision to withdraw treatment be taken). The doctor's primary responsibility, however, is to his patient's interests and not to any other individual, or to society as a whole.

The issue of obtaining assent from the relatives of incapacitated patients for medical treatment that is not life-saving has been tested in court. This has mainly related to the mentally handicapped who are unable to make decisions for themselves. Incapacitated patients are often compared to children, in that they dependent on others for most of their well-being. Although parents or guardians of children have the right to consent (or not) to medical treatment the adult mentally handicapped are in a totally different position legally. Under both English and Scottish law, the authority for parents or guardians to make decisions on behalf of another ceases when that other reaches the age of majority, regardless of that individual's ability or competence to make decisions.[19]

There have been several legal cases, both in the UK and abroad, relating to the issue of the incompetent patient and consent (usually for the mentally handicapped). These cases are brought before the courts in instances where it is felt that a certain procedure, although not life-saving, is required to cure illness or enhance the quality of the person's life.

The function of the court is to pass a proxy judgment. One way would be to attempt to decide what course of treatment the incapacitated person would have wanted, if capable of doing so. However, in all judgments the courts have stressed that the 'best interests and well-being' of the patient are paramount. This is often simple, as most people would probably prefer the chance of cure rather the prolongation of ill-health. However, this argument fails when the planned intervention is not required to treat a medical condition or does not put the patient's best interests first.[20]

An alternative is for the court to appoint some form of guardian to oversee the patient's interests. Called the 'receiver' in England and the 'curator bonis' in Scotland he has jurisdiction over the financial and business affairs of the incapacitated person but not over the person him or herself. In Scotland, the possibility of appointing a tutor-dative has been reaffirmed by the Court of Session. A tutor-dative can have control over the person so could, if within the terms of reference decided on by the Court, be able to provide proxy consent for medical treatment. One proviso is that the tutor must, at all times, act in the person's best interests.[21–23]

It would appear that none of the forms of guardianship mentioned above allows relatives to consent to the elective ventilation of a dying patient.

The unconscious patient arriving at the hospital may require urgent life-saving treatment but be unable to give consent to required therapy. The courts have recognized the defence of 'necessity' to justify taking any action necessary to save life and 'proceeding, without consent, with any procedure that it would be unreasonable, as opposed to merely inconvenient, to postpone until consent could be sought'.[18] Any treatment undertaken in the name of necessity must, again, be in the patient's best interest.

Although treating life-threatening events do not require prior consent if none is available, it appears from previous court rulings that instigating medical interventions not in the best interest of that patient are not permissible. In fact, this could leave the doctor open to the accusation of assault.

Until now, care of the organ donor did not start until after death had been diagnosed. Other patients with a fatal cerebral injury are allowed to die and to do so quickly, and with as much dignity as possible.[24] With interventional ventilation, however, actions to preserve optimal organ function for transplantation have to be started prior to death. As these procedures are not necessary for the patient's future well-being the doctor may be abandoning his responsibilities to his patient. This may be construed as assault or battery. An accusation of battery can be made following any contact by one person on another without that other's permission with no requirement to prove injury.[25] Interventional ventilation is introduced after a decision has been made that the prognosis is hopeless and no further therapeutic steps are appropriate. It would normally be acceptable to maintain patient comfort and allow nature to take its course. Continuing to treat, and especially escalating treatment, in circumstances where one would otherwise not, may be an assault. Much will depend on whether introducing artificial ventilation would have been contemplated as part of good medical practice, in the interests of the patient, had the person not been a potential organ donor (S.A.M. Maclean personal communication). Clearly, in these patients ventilation has already been excluded as a therapeutic option.

The doctrine of necessity cannot apply to interventional ventilation as the treatment may be contrary to the patient's best interests. Valid consent is not obtainable from the proposed donor and the process of dying is being prolonged with the risk of producing persistent vegetative survivors, the precise incidence of which is not known.

This problem with consent for intervention does not arise with people who currently carry a donor card because it is accepted that the donor's interests are paramount until the diagnosis of death is made, then and only then does he become a potential donor. Thus, the patient's willingness to donate his or her organs post-mortem does not influence his or her ante-mortem treatment in any way.

In law, then, the test of the best interest of the patient is all important. Patients being proposed for interventional ventilation are alive in law until they satisfy the criteria for cardiorespiratory or brainstem death. Different levels of existence between alive and dead are not recognized in law. Thus, it would appear that interventional ventilation cannot be carried out in the UK under the current legal framework. There are, however, aspects to consider other than consent.

6. Human and ICU resource considerations

Patients selected for elective ventilation will normally be cared for in an ICU, and proper care of an organ donor requires a level of care only available in the unit. Many ICUs are already short of trained nursing staff needed, with resultant complaints of overwork and low morale, and many units experiencing difficulty in recruiting new staff. Is an activity such as interventional ventilation that increases work load, especially if legally suspect, to be avoided?[26,27]

As in all aspects of health care, ICU resources are limited, indeed the UK has one of the lowest ratios of ICU to hospital beds.[28] In over 50 per cent of hospitals, patients likely to benefit from intensive care are already being refused admission due to lack of resources (beds or staff), with surgical procedures being cancelled in 48 per cent.[29] In these circumstances to expect an increase in the workload undertaken is unrealistic. Some doctors have been quoted as saying that there are not enough ICU beds for those with a chance of survival let alone for those for whom there is no hope.[30]

The presence of an electively ventilated patient delaying or stopping the admission of a patient expected to recover would be very regrettable. Discharging an interventional ventilation patient from ICU to the ward prior to death to allow admission of a 'real' patient would be very wasteful of resources and extremely upsetting to staff and relatives.

Relatives asked to 'assent' to this procedure may not really understand what is involved. Whatever is said to them, many may interpret transfer to the ICU as evidence of hope that something can be done. In the Exeter study patients suffering massive CVAs not transferred to the ICU died within 6 hours. The mean time to death in ICU for those transferred was 16.3 hours with a range of 3.3 to 41.6 hours, and indeed one patient spent 5 days in the ICU, did not 'cone', (see below) and was returned to the ward to die. This must be a distressing experience for any relative to sit to endure.

Admitting electively ventilated patients to the high dependency unit (HDU) instead of the ICU has been suggested.[31] There are two arguments against this. First, the care of the potential organ donor is becoming more sophisticated and calls for the wider use of invasive monitoring and aggressive support to optimize organ function. Second, the care of a ventilated patient requires one-to-one nursing by experienced intensive care staff to be effective.[32]

ICUs providing organs in the traditional manner are currently being reimbursed £1000 to cover the extra costs involved. This barely covers the extra costs borne by the donating unit and does not solve the problem of the shortage of beds. The active recruitment of patients for elective ventilation would leave the way open for accusations of organ selling. Indeed, four of the nine patients entered into the protocol group in Exeter did not follow the strict guidelines laid down. Had the protocol been adhered to strictly, as was supposed to happen, these patients may well have died before being available for organ donation. This disregard for the protocol in 44 per cent of cases risks bringing this new approach to organ donation into disrepute. Of greater concern is that it could adversely affect the degree of public trust in ICUs and the current organ donation scheme.

Elective ventilation has not met with the approval of the majority of ICU medical staff. The objections are based on several issues. These are: consent, commencing treatment on incapacitated patients who remain people not cadavers, prolonging the dying process for no benefit to the patient, and the unknown risk of causing harm, as well as the current shortage of ICU resources.

7. Persistent vegetative state (PVS)

Patients are selected for elective ventilation on the basis that they are expected to die anyway. Are there any detrimental effects of this procedure where the expected end-point is death? There is a possibility that interventional ventilation will prevent the evolution to brainstem death and allow the potential donor to enter a persistent vegetative state (PVS).

Brainstem death occurs due to irreversible damage to the brainstem (medulla), which connects the rest of the brain with the spinal cord. In the medulla are the areas that control respiration and cardiac activity without which survival is impossible.

The most usual final common pathway to brainstem death is hypoxia and cerebral oedema. This causes a rising intracranial pressure which presses the brainstem into the foramen magna, eventually stopping blood flow. This process is often referred to as 'coning'. Interventional ventilation introduced before, or at the time of, respiratory arrest, may interrupt this chain of events by preventing hypoxia or reducing the intracranial pressure. There is, therefore, a risk of preventing the progression to brain death despite profound brain damage having occurred. Such survivors may enter a persistent vegetative state (PVS).

PVS is a severe form of brain damage but differs from coma where the patient is unconscious and shows no reflex responses. PVS describes a group of patients who are unconscious but have cyclical patterns of sleeping and waking with eye opening. They possess reflex responses including turning towards sounds and eye following movement so giving the impression of conscious behaviour. There are, however, no signs of cerebral activity or cognitive function. All activity in the centres higher than the brainstem appear absent.

The proportion of brain-injured patients entering a PVS varies from 1 to 12 per cent of those unconscious for more than 24 hours. These patients may survive for several years, occasionally with some degree of recovery.[33] Generally, the prognosis of PVS is very poor. In fact, some have called for such patients to be allowed to die if they show no improvement after three months.[34]

For any patient initially diagnosed as being expected to die within 48 hours (as the Exeter Protocol requires) to become a PVS by unadvised intervention would be a disastrous outcome. Instead of dying, as expected, within hours this unfortunate could remain in a PVS for several years. This would be a dreadful outcome for the patient and could have a detrimental effect on the morale of the relatives, medical, and nursing staff. Together with the social and financial implications, such an outcome could also have an adverse effect on the willingness of people to become organ donors.

8. Improving the acceptability of interventional ventilation

If interventional ventilation is to be an acceptable method of procuring organs then several changes to the present scheme must be made.

The whole system of organ donation depends entirely on public goodwill. Adequate open discussion of elective ventilation of potential donors must take place. Any change or addition to the groups of people eligible to be organ donors needs to be done openly so that potential donors may discuss it with their families in advance of any cerebral event occurring. Many who are willing donors under the current system may not wish to be involved with the new. A new donor card that would allow a person to agree to interventional ventilation would be helpful if developed. Adequate public education through the media will be necessary to inform people of proposed changes. All legal and ethical dilemmas associated with interventional ventilation need open discussion and resolution by appropriate legislation if possible.

Obtaining informed consent requires that the incidence of major side-effects of any intervention or therapy is known and made available to the potential recipient. This allows the patient to weigh up the advantages against any risks involved. The incidence of PVS is not yet known so, at present, potential donors are not able to make an informed decision about interventional ventilation. An investigation into this problem has been proposed. The Potential of Interventional Ventilation in Organ Transplantation (PIVOT) study would investigate the potential for benefit from interventional ventilation versus the possibility of harm. The expected incidence of PVS is probably low or negligible therefore it may take several years to produce an accurate assessment of the risk. How low a risk is acceptable?

Whether the PIVOT study can actually be carried out legally is open to debate. Is it ethical to randomly allocate a dying incapacitated patient to a treatment group whose possible outcome is the persistent vegetative state? The patient certainly cannot consent. This coupled with the indignities related to intensive therapy (e.g. endotracheal intubation and invasive monitoring) cannot be in that patient's best interests. Furthermore, it cannot be claimed to be necessary for the patient. Is the defence that society needs the information for the future strong enough?

If at all possible, the risk of PVS needs to be explored so that a realistic forecast of risk may be offered. Thus, the PIVOT study should be completed before any further expansion of the protocol is undertaken. However, as already stated it is doubtful whether this study could legally take place. In the event of PVS occurring the accepted mode of withdrawing therapy needs to be clarified. At present, the British Medical Association guidelines recommend continuing support for a minimum of 12 months. Do the courts need to be involved in every case before the withdrawal of support?

Some have called for PVS survivors to be allowed to die if they show no signs of recovery. The recent case of Anthony Bland may have set a precedent for the withdrawal of treatment and so allowing persistent vegetative survivors to die. Mr Bland was a 17-year-old victim of the Hillsborough disaster in April 1989 where he suffered hypoxic brain damage such that he existed in a persistent vegetative state from then until 1993 with no sign of recovery.[35] The request to withdraw all supportive therapy from Mr Bland was made on the grounds that it was in his, although not necessarily in society's, best interest.

Although the Law Lords judgment in agreement has been heralded as a breakthrough in the care of the chronically brain-injured, they stated that the Bland case did not, in fact, set a precedent and all future cases would require to seek a declaration from the court.[36] This judgment thus does not set a precedent for the treatment of, or the removal of treatment from PVS patients in the future.

With the law as it presently stands the adequacy of consent obtained on behalf of an incapacitated patient is uncertain. The Law Commission is currently investigating the whole issue of consent, especially concerning the incapacitated patient.[37] The use of advance directives (or living wills) from the patient has been suggested. Advance directives are in common use in the US for specifying treatments that the patient is willing, or not, to receive. They are beginning to appear in the UK. If introduced for interventional ventilation they would allow more 'real' consent to be obtained as the person would have had to think about the possibility well in advance.

A criticism of advance directives is that they may prohibit treatment that will be highly effective in a particular set of circumstances. For example, a refusal to allow renal dialysis would preclude this even for renal failure judged to be short term and reversible, so the advance directive may actually act against the patient's best interests. Conversely, others are so poorly worded as the be of no guidance to the medical staff as to the person's wishes. The Terence Higgins Trust has designed an advance directive specifically for patients suffering from the terminal stages of AIDS. Being designed for a single disease process it is much less likely to accidentally act against the patient. A similar document could be drafted to cover intracerebral events and interventional ventilation but would not interfere with the active treatment of survivable conditions.

The King's Fund Institute recently published a report on ways to improve the supply of donor organs for transplantation.[38] In discussing the elective ventilation of dying patients they identified two main objections. The first is the issue of consent which under the current legal situation cannot be granted. If this procedure is to be continued or expanded then its legal status will require to be clarified by statute. It will need to be accepted that society's need for potential donors allows the introduction of a procedure patently not in the patient's best interests. The main ethical argument against interventional ventilation is the possibility of producing patients in a persistent vegetative state. As already stated the legality of the PIVOT study to investigate the risk of PVS is in doubt and it has been postponed.

9. Conclusion

The elective ventilation of dying patients until brainstem death occurs is a proposed method of procuring organs for transplantation. If carried out on a national scale it might meet the UK's requirements for kidneys and greatly improve the supply of other organs. However, the criticisms of interventional ventilation are both legal and ethical. Consent for interventional ventilation cannot be obtained from the potential donor. Even if changes are made to the donor card or advanced directives are used, proper informed consent is impossible to obtain. This is because the risk of PVS, the major potential harm, cannot be forecast at the moment. Although investigation of this is planned the legality of the investigation is also questioned.

Delaying a dying patient's death, and the risk of causing PVS, in order to harvest organs later are the main ethical objections. Using scarce intensive care resources for ventilating dying patients when there is a real possibility of this preventing another patient access to the ICU is unacceptable. Not only could it adversely affect another patient but it would be demoralizing for the staff.

Interventional ventilation is not the only alternative to the present practice for organ retrieval. More effort needs to be made to enrol the 6 per cent of ICU patients in whom organ donation is not considered. The current refusal rate of almost 30 per cent needs to be addressed, and it may be that an opt-out scheme, as used in many European countries, should be considered. The use of non-heart-beating donors whose kidneys are rapidly cooled immediately after death has recently been reported. This is legally and ethically more acceptable, as no intervention is performed until the patient is declared dead. It is not, however, an alternative source for organs other than kidneys at this stage.[39,40]

Over-enthusiastic adoption of elective ventilation of dying patients for organ retrieval before the public fully understands the procedures may lead to criticism. Worse still, it could cause a loss of confidence in the transplant programme. Legal obstacles could be cleared by changing legislation but ethical objections may not be solved so easily. Certainly, until a further discussion of legal and ethical aspects is undertaken, more resources are made available, and the public adequately educated, further promotion of interventional ventilation appears unwise.

Note added in proof

Since this chapter was originally written the Government has taken legal advice as to the legality of interventional ventilation. They have been advised that in all probability interventional ventilation is illegal, so in September 1994 announced that all such programmes should cease. There continues to be active debate of the issues in the medical press. It is to hoped that public debate and consultation will follow and allow a final decision about the future of interventional ventilation to be made.[41]

The Law Commission document concerning medical treatment and mental incapacity suggested that advance directives could be used to refuse treatment. The Commission was of the opinion that advance consent to treatment not in the patient's best interest would not render that treatment lawful.[42]

Notes

1. Wing, A.J. and Chang, R.W.S. (1994). Non-heart beating donors as a source of kidneys. *British Medical Journal*, 308, 549–10.

2. Younger, S.J. and Arnold, R.M. (1993). Ethical, psychosocial, and public policy implications of procuring organs from non-heart beating cadaver donors. *Journal of the American Medical Association*, 269, 2769–74.
3. UK Transplant Service (1989). *Annual Report*. UK Transplant Service, Bristol.
4. Feest, T.G., *et al.* (1990). Protocol for increasing organ donation after cerebro-vascular deaths in a district general hospital. *Lancet*, 335, 1133–5.
5. Riad, H. (1993). Elective ventilation for organ donation. *British Journal of Hospital Medicine*, 50, 438–42.
6. Wakeford, R.E. and Stepney, R. (1989). Obstacles to organ donation. *British Journal of Surgery*, 76, 435–9.
7. Gore, S.M., Cable, D.J., and Holland, A.J. (1992). Organ donation from intensive care units in England and Wales: Two year confidential audit of deaths in intensive care. *British Medical Journal*, 304, 349–55.
8. Gore, S.M., Hinds, C.J., and Rutherford, A.J. (1989). Organ donation from intensive care units in England. *British Medical Journal*, 299, 1193–7.
9. Bodenham, A., Berridge, J.C., and Park, G.R. (1989). Brain stem death and organ donation. *British Medical Journal*, 299, 1009–10.
10. Dennis, M.J.S., Ryan, M.J., and Blamey, R.W. (1989). Brain stem death and organ donation. *British Medical Journal*, 299, 1218.
11. Collins, C.H. (1992). Elective ventilation for organ donation—the case in favour. *Care of the Critically Ill*, 8, 57–9.
12. Bates, R. (1992). Doctors dilemma on donor ethics. *Hospital Doctor*, 30 April, 30.
13. Mason, J.K. and McCall Smith, R.A. (ed.) (1991). Declaration of Helsinki (Revised 1975). Introduction. In *Law and medical ethics*, Appx F, (4th edn), p. 447. Butterworths, London.
14. BMA (British Medical Association) (1993). *Medical ethics today*, p. 28. BMJ Publishing Group, London.
15. Conference of Medical Royal Colleges and their Faculties in the UK (1976). Diagnosis of brain death. *British Medical Journal*, 2, 1187–8.
16. Conference of Medical Royal Colleges and their Faculties in the UK (1979). Diagnosis of brain death. *British Medical Journal*, i, 3320.
17. Nicholls, A. and Riad, H. (1993). Organ donation. *British Medical Journal*, 306, 517.
18. Brazier, M. (1992). *Medicine, patients and the law*, (2nd edn), p. 91. Penguin. London.
19. Walker, D.M. (1988). *Principles of Scots Private Law*, (4th edn), p. 219. Clarendon Press, Oxford.
20. McLean, S.A.M. (1989). *A patient's right to know: Information disclosure, the doctor and the law*, pp. 63–68. Dartmouth, Aldershot.
21. Note 19, pp. 316–17.
22. Note 13, p. 282.
23. Ward, A.D. (1987). Revival of tutors-dative. *Scottish Legal Times*, 69.
24. Park, G.R., Gunning, K.E., Lindop, M.J., and Roe, P.G. (1993). Organ donation. *British Medical Journal*, 306, 145.
25. Note 13, p. 238.
26. Routh, G. (1992). Elective ventilation for organ donation—the case against. *Care of the Critically Ill*, 8, 60–1.

27. Willats, S. (1994). Elective ventilation. *British Journal of Hospital Medicine*, 51, 450–1.
28. Lavery, G.G., Lowry, K.G., Johnston, J.R., Coppel, D.L. (1993). Organ donation. *British Medical Journal*, 306, 517.
29. The Royal College of Anaesthetists (1994). *National ITU audit 1992/1993*. p. 6. London.
30. Ballantyne, A. (1990). Patient at the brink of death being kept alive for transplants. *Sunday Times*, 18 March, p. 7.
31. Williams, R. (1993). More donor organs for transplantation. Elective ventilation proposals. *Journal of the Royal College of Physicians of London*, 27, 214–15.
32. Searle, J.F. (1989). Organs for transplantation. *British Medical Journal*, 299, 1464.
33. Andrews, K. (1993). Recovery of patients after four months or more in the persistent vegetative state. *British Medical Journal*, 306, 1597–9.
34. Jennet, B. and Dyer, C. (1991). Persistent vegetative state and the right to die: the United States and Britain. *British Medical Journal*, 302, 1256–8.
35. *Airedale NHS Trust v. Bland* [1993] 2 WLR 316.
36. Dyer, C. (1993). Law lords rule that Tony Bland does not create precedent. *British Medical Journal*, 306, 413–14.
37. Law Commission Paper No. 129.
38. New, W., *et al.* (1994). *A question of give and take*. The King's Fund Institute, London.
39. Varty, K., *et al.* (1993). Response to organ retrieval programme using non-heart beating donors. *British Medical Journal*, 308, 575.
40. Phillips, A.O., *et al.* (1993). Renal grafts from non-heart beating donors. *British Medical Journal*, 308, 575–6.
41. Riad, H. and Nicholls, A. (1995). An ethical debate: Elective ventilation of potential organ donors. *British Medical Journal*, 310, 714–18.
42. The Law Commission (1995). *Mental incapacity*, p. 70. HMSO, London.

11

Rational Resource Allocation: Management Perspectives

Roger Dyson

1. Introduction

The demand for health care now exceeds supply in the public health care system of every developed country in the world. Every country responds by rationing and only the rationing systems differ; in their crudeness or sophistication, and in their approach. There is a general perception that rationing is becoming tighter as the result of a greater imbalance of supply and demand, but no evidence is advanced in this review for this surmise and technically it is not essential for the analysis or the conclusions. This chapter will look at demand and supply issues at both the macro- and the micro-levels of health care provision, and the micro-level case study will be the provision of intensive care services.

2. A model for analysing health care demand

In the UK it has been fashionable to analyse the supply side of health care delivery. In 1974, there was a major reorganization in the delivery of health care and the definition was extended to include all previous local authority services, with the exception of personal social services. In 1977, arrangements were made to separate public from private medicine within National Health Service (NHS) institutions. In 1980, the organizational hierarchy of the NHS was reduced and in 1984, following the Griffiths' Report, the managerial control of NHS resources was tightened. The most radical reorganization took place in 1990 and introduced purchaser/provider contracting as one of a number of means of creating a managed market to keep the costs of health care under control by competition. What unites these and other initiatives since 1948 is that they have had as their driving force the objective of using NHS resources more effectively (i.e. getting more health care per pound sterling provided).

This supply-side approach has always been more attractive to politicians of all parties than either recognizing that greater demand requires greater resources pro rata, or by tackling demand itself. Few people would argue, other than hypothetically, that the UK or any other developed country can match increases in demand pro rata with resources. It follows that supply is fairly inflexible in the short and medium term, and it can be argued that demand is the more dynamic variable of the two and it is by analysing demand that we are likely to achieve the most rational allocation of resources. The model below analyses demand on three levels: potential, expressed, and realized.

Potential demand. This is concerned exclusively with known and scientifically proven services and therapies. The key assumption that underlies this demand-side analysis is that potential demand for known services and therapies could already consume the whole of the gross national product (GNP), if all potentially benefiting patients came forward and demanded the full range of all available services. To précis a longer discussion, this might involve the provision of unlimited intensive care, the widespread availability of cardiac arrest teams to patients deemed to be at high risk outside the hospital, and the international purchase of donor organs for transplant, etc. Even if patients demanded the less dramatic services that would benefit them, the potential scale of that request alone would swamp the existing NHS services.

Expressed demand. This is merely that element of potential demand which patients have already come forward to request; very largely via their general practitioner.

Realized demand. This is a proxy for supply. In any period of time it measures the amount of expressed demand that has been met with an appropriate supply.

Because demand exceeds supply there will be a gap in any period of time between the extent of expressed demand and the extent of realized demand or supply. Politicians frequently use the concept of the waiting list to measure this gap and this now includes a measurement of both in-patient and out-patient waiting lists. These waiting lists are themselves a proxy for a much more complex range of contributors to the gap. The general practitioner diverts many types of demand that could easily find their way forward to the measurable queues, and in hospitals consultants constantly take decisions not to provide additional services that could be provided.

At times when the gap between expressed and realized demand appears to remain constant, there is less controversy about the NHS. It is during periods when the gap is rising that the future and organization of the NHS is a matter for major political argument and debate. The gap widens because of an increase in expressed demand in excess of the government's willingness or ability to increase realized demand. It is therefore a matter of considerable importance to determine why expressed demand continues to grow (i.e. why there is a continual leakage from potential to expressed demand). In a chapter of this length a more complex debate can be summarized under a number of broad headings.

Demographic change.   Given assumptions about the greater annual consumption of resources by the more elderly part of the population, any shift in the balance of the population towards the higher-age cohorts is of itself likely to increase expressed demand. This is happening at the present time, although there is a debate about its extent based on the different age ranges measured. The government gestures towards demographic change by including a percentage allocation for this purpose in the annual funding of the NHS. In recent years, this has been set at 1 per cent but no research has been undertaken to justify the relevance or suitability of this allocation. There are grounds for believing that 1 per cent on the total NHS budget is a considerable underestimate of the full effect of demographic change because of lengthening life-expectancy and the concentration of health care expenditure in the very last year of life. It is not possible to reach a firm conclusion on the extent of the contribution made by demographic change to the growth of expressed demand because there has never been the necessary research.

Social attitudes.   Changes in social attitudes are even less easy to measure. The main arguments are that the current generation now regard health care as a right rather than a privilege. There is certainly much more public awareness of health care issues and the media constantly focus on health care opportunities, which in turn substantially encourages a switch from potential to expressed demand. A more secular society is more concerned with living longer in this life than with preparing for the next, and perhaps partially for these reasons we have become a much less pain-tolerant society with far greater demands on pain relief. That these changes in society contribute to the transfer from potential to expressed demand is undeniable, but the extent of the contribution has not been measured.

Supply-induced demand.   Perhaps the most important long-term factor is the implication of supply-induced demand. Very simply, stated it means that for each new scientific and skill development, whether of electronic technology, complex drug structures, or surgical techniques and body tissue replacements, the availability of a new service will create a demand in excess of the ability to meet that demand. In terms of the model, supply-induced demand carries with it the implication that expressed demand will rise by greater than realized demand and thus add to the overall burden of rationing.

Such an argument is hard for clinicians. There have been major developments in the history of medical science where a new technology or new drug has substantially reduced an element of expressed demand and narrowed the gap. The defeat of tuberculosis would be an obvious illustration and there are others including a range of infectious diseases. Alas, across the totality of health care provision, the phenomenon of supply-induced demand has contributed to a continuing rise in the gap and one has only to think of the implication in the 21st century of the ability, one by one, to replace the organs of the body with more effective artificial substitutes.

At the national level there is now an unspoken fear that substantial investment in medical research will only add to the pressures on the NHS, and it is not insignificant in this context that public investment in medico-scientific research has been declining across the world as a percentage of GNP. Politicians are turning to increasingly low-technology policies for fear of the consequence of supply-induced demand. NHS ministers can urge us to swim as an alternative therapy to drugs for high blood pressure, and, more seriously, the introduction of Medisave in Singapore seven years ago constituted a dramatic switch from building more high-technology hospitals with the transfer of resources into local clinics, all equipped with basic theatres and offering no wider range of more sophisticated services.

3. Macro-level initiatives

Against a background of rationing, politicians, clinicians, and health economists have sought strategies to make the most effective use of the available resource. Two such initiatives are selected here as they constitute illustrations of two very different approaches to the question of how to make the best use of available resources.

The Oregon experiment[1]

The State of Oregon in the US decided to allow the population to ballot for their priorities from a range of available health care services in order to help politicians determine the relative allocation of resources between these services. The Bush Administration held up the Oregon experiment on the grounds that it infringed the rights of minorities not to be discriminated against, but the Clinton Administration seems set to allow the experiment to go forward. It is an attempt to allow the population to have ownership of the rationing decisions in order to minimize the potential hostility to rationing. It raises innumerable ethical issues that are not pursued in this chapter.

The implication of Oregon is that certain sections of clinical demand might not receive any public funding according to public response. A variant of this exists within the purchaser/provider arrangements of the present-day NHS. Purchasing authorities are required to assess the health care needs of the population relative to the resource available and to make the necessary arrangements for purchasing services from providers to meet those needs. This gives purchasers the right to define the services for which they will or will not contract. Examples exist today of purchasers deciding not to buy a number of surgical procedures, such as tattoo removal and vasectomy reversal, not buying hydrotherapy services for NHS patients, and more controversially in one or two cases, indicating their refusal to buy *in vitro* fertilization. It can be argued that this element of the recent NHS reforms contains within it some element of demand-side control, but the controversy there has already been over the issue of purchasing *in vitro* fertilization indicates how limited the powers of the purchasers really are in this respect.

The strength of the Oregon experiment lies in the democratic underpinning of the electoral process. The weakness of the purchaser's position in the UK lies in the public perception that it is merely an arbitrary decision by bureaucrats.

Quality-adjusted life-years (QUALYs)[2]

This particular form of quality of life measure was developed at York University and represents an attempt to measure the quality adjusted life years as a basis for allocating resources between different health care services. It is important for this analysis to note that whilst it is possible to try to measure QUALYs within a medical specialty, the prime purpose of the analysis is to undertake broader measures of quality adjusted life years between specialties to determine their relative allocation of resources.

Both of these approaches attempt to make the best use of the available resource by directing demand, but they do not attempt to tackle the broader question of the causes of the rise in the level of expressed demand. This is returned to in the conclusion.

4. Micro-level analysis applied to intensive care

In the attempt to get the best use out of the resource of an intensive care unit (ICU), there seem to be two separate areas for debate.

Who should be admitted to intensive care and for how long?

The literature seems to agree that survivors are not only preferable to non-survivors but that they also cost less per day of intensive care. 'Patients with a chance of survival of less than 50 per cent incurred costs that were twice as high as those with a chance of survival of over 50 per cent'.[3] Alternatively, '. . . we then examined the relations between this prognosis, the actual outcome, and the resource expenditure during the single hospitalization. We found that the care of non-survivors involved a significantly higher mean expenditure than did the care of survivors'.[4] This conclusion would be extremely helpful if it could be determined in advance who would be the survivors, but attempts to determine in advance who will survive have not produced unanimous conclusions. APACHE II scores may be a good predictor of the first day's costs, thus '. . . the cost of the first day of management was significantly related to the APACHE II score and individual costs on the first day may be predicted from admission APACHE II scores'.[3] However, there seems little or no agreement that APACHE II is an adequate predictor of survival or non-survival. Even though it could be argued that, '... patients who died on the ITU had significantly higher APACHE II scores ... and there was no significant variation in the distribution of the patients' age or duration of admission',[3] this result could not be the final arbiter because of the existence of patients who survived despite higher APACHE II scores. Equally, the extent of organ failure, or the number of ventilated days provided, may be a good predictor but an insufficient one to judge access to or discharge from an ICU.

For example, Wagner examined 227 patients who were ventilated for more than seven days and noted that these patients consumed 37 per cent of the total ITU resources but represented only 12 per cent of all ventilated patients and 6 per cent of all ITU admissions. Furthermore, 21 per cent of the 37 per cent of total resource consumption occurred after the seventh day of ventilatory support.[5]

The value of these and other cost–benefit studies is considerable but seems to lie more in enabling diagnoses to be put in rank order than in taking immediate decisions about which type of patients should have the right of access to intensive care and which should not. There is an understandable reluctance in the clinical research to reach judgements about the total exclusion of any category of patient, although it seems clear that the attempts to get the best use of intensive care resources for the patients that use them will continue, if only to maximize total patient benefit.

Attempts to measure the subsequent quality of life of discharged survivors are relevant to the debate in so far as the information assists clinicians in judging who should access intensive care beds in the first place. The difficulty in achieving quality of life measurements is partly due to the fact that success for an intensive care clinician seems so often to be measured in terms of survival from the immediate crisis rather than in terms of the longer-term prognosis. Perhaps this is partly due to the fact that the intensive care clinician passes the patient back to the admitting clinican who is then subsequently responsible for clinical management and possible hospital discharge. To be fair to the intensive care clinician, he or she receives a patient with the overt or implicit instruction to overcome the immediate crisis and intensivists can be forgiven for focusing in a single-minded way on the immediate objective. This raises interesting questions about the objectives of the admitting clinicians who hand over their patients, but this is beyond the framework of this chapter.

The increasing debate about resource allocation has, however, caused intensive care clinicians to focus upon quality of life issues where their case is inevitably not strong because of the relatively poor prognosis of many survivors. What is more, attempts to justify intensive care expenditure *per se* on the basis of the quality of life of survivors seem flawed. If they do not measure the quality of life gain available from the next alternative use of the resource, for example, would the provision of *in vitro* fertilization with the same resource produce a better overall quality of life for the totality of patients? This brings us back to the York University's QUALYs and the macro-level debate.

How many intensive care beds do we need?

Inevitably, this debate takes its stand on the potential number of patients who could benefit from access to intensive care beds if more were available. It is a debate that is inevitably subjective as it pleads for a specialty without attempting any broader cost–benefit analysis. Specifying the number of intensive care beds required for X hospital beds or for X thousand of the population is about as legitimate as renal physicians demanding more continuous ambulatory peritoneal dialysis (i.e. the demand is there so we should have the resource to fill it). This comment is not meant to be critical of the argument itself, because the role of the person(s) involved in balancing the available resource between services is to be as informed as possible about the level of demand. This approach should not, however, lead its advocates into belief that the ever-changing ratio is some statistically accurate analysis based on a clear and finite identification of demand. It merely reflects what medical science is capable of achieving at a given point in time and is special pleading from one specialty rather than another.

5. Mechanisms for access to intensive care

Whatever the ethical problems in making choices about individual patients there has, is, and always will be a mechanism for determining the availability of intensive care beds in a national health care system. There are really only two alternatives: purchaser contracts and rigid criteria for access.

Purchaser contracts

In today's NHS it is for the purchaser to buy intensive care beds within the negotiation of annual contracts. This also applies to high dependency units (HDUs). Within the resources available to the purchaser it will require money to be committed to maintain and staff a given number of beds. Within the 12 months of the contract the provider will have no additional beds or resources. Once this framework has been set, it will be for the skill of the staff to set and change the criteria for admission and discharge as determined by the daily demand for beds. When the pressure of demand is high, criteria will have to be very strict, and when demand happens to dip, criteria may be less strict—and it will be for the clinical staff in charge of the unit to determine sensitive changes to the strength of the criteria as demand peaks and troughs.

This is not an attractive prospect for clinicians who feel that they are being made personally responsible for resolving ethical dilemmas that have an economic origin. It is possible for an extra contractual referral (ECR) or transfer to be made from one overcrowded intensive care unit to another. This implies that the purchasing authority will meet an additional bill for intensive care over and above its contract commitment to the referring ICU.

At first, purchasing authorities sought to delay such transfers by the requirement of permission, but as the result of pressure on politicians, emergency ECRs have been allowed in advance of financial permission. This seemed to offer clinicians in charge of ICUs a way out of the more agonizing dilemmas. Inevitably, however, this route is now being closed as purchasing authorities agree contracts with one another for intensive care transfers to be handled on a 'knock for knock' basis. This means that hospital A with intensive care beds may transfer one emergency patient to the ICU of hospital B, and that this will entitle hospital B to make a transfer back to the ICU of hospital A; each transfer being balanced out within the original contracts of the two purchasing authorities. In other words, a health care system with finite resources cannot afford to open a blank cheque for intensive care and has always to seek to circumvent clinicians' attempts to free themselves from the constraint.

Rigid criteria for access

If clinicians ever decide to refuse responsibility for this moral juggling act then financial control, inescapable with finite resources, would resort to rigid criteria for access and rigid procedures. The judgement of clinicians would be replaced by a series of strict and inflexible rules for access based on APACHE II scores, or on simple rules based on organ failure, or on rules that stipulated the maximum number of ventilated days to be made available to an NHS patient. The first two of these would be easier to operate because they limit access to intensive care beds, the last would be more difficult because it would involve removing a patient from ventilation who *might* have survived. It would not, of course, be possible to take a patient off a ventilator in an arbitrary fashion without clinical justification, *unless* there was a clear and pre-established protocol which all patients knew and to which all patients, and the relatives of children under the age of 18, subscribed as part of their consent to treatment at the start of the process.

The first of these options, rather than the second, describes the current state of affairs in NHS intensive care. It is to the benefit of patients and the credit of the medical profession that this is so. Clinicians' frustrations with having to play God can be understood, but then nobody chose to be an intensive care specialist without knowing that this was a consequence. No politician will ever take personal responsibility and it is probably fortunate for society that this is so. There would be many adverse consequences for a society in which politicians *were* prepared to take personal responsibility for withdrawing life from individual citizens. If a crisis were to occur in the future, politicians always have the Oregon option as a means of limiting intensive care expenditure. The under-fives, or even the under-eighteens benefit, in terms of access to intensive care, but any voting system would probably leave the elderly well outside the current level of access. Would this make it any easier for clinicians to initiate the consequences of any public decision to restrict access? I doubt it.

6. Conclusion

The painful conclusion of this line of reasoning is that the resource argument will always dominate the clinical argument in the provision of any single clinical service. Once a finite resource has been set for a service within the year, clinicians struggle to exercise the most effective and the fairest clinical judgements about service access and treatment. Those who find the clinical judgements and ethical problems too distressing will either leave intensive medicine or will never enter it. In just the same way not every doctor is suited to the responsibility of a surgeon to go into the theatre and fail, and go back again the next day to risk failure again.

In a public health care system that is anxious to avoid supply-induced demand implications intensive care specialists can only go to the purchasers of health care and seek, by whatever means possible, to negotiate bit by bit for one extra bed here and one extra bed there. Anguish about the ethical dilemma may persuade some purchasers some of the time, but the renal physicians of the early 1980s overplayed their hand and encouraged a deep cynicism about 'shroud-waving' which has worked to their disadvantage since. Clinicians in intensive care should not be tempted to overstate their case in the same way.

Notes

1. Brookings Institute (1991, December). *Rationing America's medical care: The Oregon Plan and beyond.* The Brookings Institute, Washington, DC.
2. Williams, A. (1985). Economics of coronary artery bypass grafting. *British Medical Journal,* 291, 326–9.
3. Ridley, S., Biggam, M., and Stone, P. (1993). A cost–benefit analysis of intensive therapy. *Anaesthesia,* 48, 14–19.
4. Allean, S., *et al.* (1981). Prognosis, survival, and the expenditure of hospital resources for patients in an intensive care unit. *New England Journal of Medicine,* 305, 667.
5. Ridley, S. (1993). Cost and outcome of intensive care. *Current Anaesthesia and Critical Care,* 4, 204–7.

12
Rational Resource Allocation: Ethical Perspectives

Lesley McTurk

1. Introduction

Of the many complex ethical issues encountered by those working in an intensive care unit (ICU), the one of rational allocation of resources can seem the most difficult. Central to this issue is the decision of whether to commence or continue treatment, and the problem of withdrawing or 'switching off' life support.

Major surgical procedures can depend on a post-operative period in the intensive care unit, as a routine part of patient recovery. Open heart surgery is one example, and meeting the need for such operations is dependent on sufficient beds being available in the ICU. This means there must be a flow through of patients who leave the unit and do not 'block' the beds for extended periods of time. The allocation of scarce resources within the ICU begins with appropriate admission to intensive care; but it also includes premature discharge of patients to accommodate new admissions; admitting patients to alternative wards when no intensive care beds are available; and the withholding and withdrawing of life support to make room in the unit for other patients.[1]

There are, of course, other levels of allocation that impact on the availability of intensive care. The overall budget allocated to health in a publicly funded system, and at the intermediate level, between hospitals and specialties, are resource allocation decisions affecting all areas of health care. Other issues arising in the ICU can also have implications for the allocation of resources, relating to resuscitation, organ transplantation, and the criteria for brain death, raising their own ethical concerns in addition to those of allocation.

This chapter focuses on decisions to withhold and to withdraw treatment, and the question of when it is ethical to 'switch off' life support, in the context of scarcity of resources. Removing the patient from such support is often quite appropriate. It may no longer be required, the patient having recovered sufficiently to cope on his or her own; or the patient may have deteriorated to the extent that brain death has occurred so that he or she will gain no further benefit from continuing treatment.

Effective management of resources in the ICU requires detailed information about outcome, yet little is available. The demand for intensive care is increasing and with it the need to optimize the use of resources in these units. Such pressures heighten the need for a rational and informed approach to resource management. Assumptions such as the more severe the illness the greater the demand for treatment and care, need to be questioned. Decisions in the ICU can involve that most difficult compromise, between sustaining life itself for one patient, and enhancing the quality of life of others.

As well as such compromises, resource allocation decisions can involve conflicts of interest, and of particular concern are decisions made to limit therapy or withdraw support in the face of the family requesting continued care. An example is when the health care team recommends a DNR (do not resuscitate) order but the relatives want 'everything done'. What is the extent and nature of the duty of physicians to defer to family wishes, especially when those wishes are unrealistic? Similar issues arise where it is the patient him or herself who requests 'inappropriate' treatment, although this is not complicated by the added problem of having to weigh the dignity and integrity of the patient against the psychological benefits to the family gained from pursuing further invasive yet futile treatment.

Relatives may also request that treatment be withdrawn inappropriately. This raises ethical issues regarding the autonomy of the patient, whether the relatives are proper proxies for the patient, and the duty of the physician to act in the patient's best interests even if this means overriding the wishes of the relatives. However, it does not have the same implications for resource allocation as when treatment is requested, and this is the concern of this chapter.

2. 'Futile' care

Allocation of resources in the ICU will often depend on what is meant by the term 'futile' care, as it is on this basis that treatment may be justifiably withdrawn. There can be no obligation on the doctor to provide care that will not benefit the patient. Similarly, there is no obligation to receive such treatment: if the patient feels that care will provide no benefit they, or their proxies, have the right to refuse treatment, even if refusal leads to death. The well-known case of Karen Ann Quinlan helped establish this principle.[2]

As a result of a car accident while in her twenties, Karen Ann Quinlan was left in a persistent vegetative state, technically called 'brain dead'. A mechanical ventilator was used to keep her alive. After seven months her parents went to court to obtain an order for the hospital to remove her from the ventilator, against counter-arguments that this would be tantamount to murder. The court recognized the general right of competent people to refuse treatment, or for a proxy to make treatment decisions on behalf of an incompetent person, and authorized the removal. Karen Ann Quinlan proved able to breathe for herself and did not die for another nine years; but the principle behind this case remains, of the right to refuse treatment, either by the patient or her proxy.

It is when treatment is requested which may be medically futile that ethical questions are most acutely raised. One reason care may be futile is because providing care may have no demonstrable effect, at a chosen level of probability. Understood narrowly, 'medical treatment is futile if it cannot produce its physiological effect'.[3] Doctors will be best placed to judge such effects as they are based on clinical indicators. However, treatment may be futile in another sense: when even though it produces a positive physiological effect, it produces no net benefit. This is the case when the burdens of care such as pain, distress, and poor prognosis outweigh the benefits. Here, the doctor and the patient (or their relatives) may disagree over the balance of benefits and burdens that the treatment offers, weighing them up differently. The term 'medically futile' is unhelpful in this context as it does not reflect such distinctions, glossing over the psychological benefits and the fact that personal, religious, or even societal benefit may accrue from care—even in the absence of 'medical benefit'.

The ambiguity of the term 'futile' arises from its interpretation within different parameters, and can cause problems. Treatment which is physiologically futile (i.e. does not produce the sought after effect: no 'medical benefit') needs to be distinguished from care that is not futile in this sense, but nevertheless has no *net* benefit. Clearly, if treatment will do no good it seems senseless to provide it, and doctors are absolved of any obligation to do so. Ethical guidelines state that, 'a treatment that cannot be reasonably expected to achieve even its physiological objective is physiologically futile and need not be offered or provided if requested'. They further state that, 'doctors are not obliged to provide physiologically futile treatments (i.e. treatments that cannot produce the desired physiological change)'.[4]

Yet equally clearly, the question remains of who is to balance the benefits and burdens, where some benefits are not wholly within the province of medical expertise. There is also the question of who is the appropriate judge of risk: the doctor may judge the probability of success such as to make the treatment not worth pursuing, but the patient or their surrogate may view the same probability differently.

In cases where *net* benefit must be assessed, it can be argued that doctors are not best placed to balance the benefits and burdens, as they have no special expertise where non-physiological benefits are concerned. There are cases where the patient (or their relatives) believes the treatment would be beneficial, but in the judgement of the doctor the treatment is 'futile' in this broader sense: that the burdens would far outweigh the benefits.

Thus, although the treatment may not be physiologically futile, it may have consequences for the patient that the medical profession deems unacceptable, such as mutilation, pain, or loss of function. Alternatively, while again the treatment may not be physiologically futile, the majority of people may deem the consequences unacceptable. (The shift in public attitude to maintaining permanently comatose patients on respirators may be illustrative here.[4]

When patients (or their proxies) request care that in the opinion of the medical staff is futile (no *net* benefit), we see a conflict between what might be seen as the squandering of scarce resources (and consequently other needy patients being deprived of benefits), and the right of patients to medical treatment. Is there an overriding of patients' autonomy if such care is denied? Veatch points out that the principle of autonomy does not automatically give patients the right of access to care.[5] If it did, patients would be entitled to demand and receive quack therapies from their doctors, such as laetrile.[6] However the right of access to health care may be justified by reference to other principles, of justice, or even beneficence.

When the doctor and the patient have a difference of opinion regarding treatment and outcome, this may be based on their differing values and attitudes to risk. In the case of Karen Ann Quinlan, the assessment of benefit from the viewpoint of the patient's family took precedence over the clinician's judgement about medical benefits for the patient. However, the continuing treatment of Karen Ann Quinlan did not have an opportunity cost in terms of benefits forgone by other needy patients, due to the structure of the US health care system, where resources are not limited providing payment is made.

When requests are made for treatment which the doctor believes have no net benefit but where the patient disagrees, or where there are 'unusual tastes in medical services',[7] or when a treatment is demanded where the cost is high but the benefit marginal, who should be the judge as to whether scarce resources are used? Given the burdens imposed on others by such requests, who may have stronger moral claims on resources, these parties will surely have an interest in the sorts of decisions made, and who they should be made by. We have already said that doctors have no special expertise in balancing the benefits where they are not exclusively medical (physiological). However, they are in a special position by virtue of their relationship with the patient and family, and possibly their experience of similar situations.

We are reminded here that no decisions in medicine are value-free, even those based on so-called scientific or technical 'facts'. All are based on a shaping and sifting of data, choice of language, and selection of conceptual frameworks for evaluation. The belief system and values of the researcher, the scientist, the clinician—and to some extent the patient—all inform the clinical decision. So, even the doctor's judgement regarding the physiological futility of treatment may be value-laden.

The doctors' duty to act in the best interests of their patients can conflict with their duty to protect society's interests. The resulting tension is persistent in discussions about resource allocation in health care. Although doctors clearly have a duty to the patient in front of them, if the exercise of this duty is seen frequently to override society's interests then inevitably others (governments, managers, bureaucrats, or the law) will need to step in and curtail the activities of doctors; in other words, to limit their clinical freedom in some way. Yet codifying the process of medical decision-making in clinical protocols, and especially in statutory law, has far-reaching consequences.[8]

A traditional way of describing the responsibility of the medical profession towards patients maintains that the doctor's duty is to do everything for the individual patient, irrespective of cost. But there is an alternative perspective, perhaps more controversial, where the doctor's duty to the individual patient is assessed in the context of society's rights and needs:

This requires the physician to consider the care to be provided in terms of the fair allocation of resources. To such physicians the issues are social and ethical as well as economic and medical.[9]

This alternative perspective on medical responsibility for the resource consequences of clinical decisions sees the profession's active consideration of the opportunity cost of resource use as complementary to their clinical freedom, rather than necessarily infringing it. It implies, 'acceptance of responsibility for the care of individual patients and for the consequent alteration in the availability of health care to others—the opportunity cost'.[9]

When resources are scarce, or when demand outstrips supply, there will be health services to which the patient has no claim in equity. Under such conditions, provision of futile or unnecessary care may violate the rights of those with a stronger moral claim to resources. Taking a responsible attitude to resource allocation means attempting to articulate what services (or what levels of services) will be provided, and to whom, with relevant criteria being defined. A notable attempt to achieve this was in Oregon,[10] which began with the decision to withdraw funding from all transplants (heart, liver, pancreas, bone marrow) under the Medicaid programme, in order to extend basic health care to the women and children in the state who were uninsured. Other countries are moving towards a definition of core services which will be accessible on affordable terms to all, or publicly funded, although such attempts are fraught with difficulties.[11]

In the light of this, we should look at what the objective of the intensive care unit is. Professor G. R. Dunstan makes the following observation:

The success of intensive care is not . . . to be measured only by the statistics of survival, as though each death were a medical failure. It is to be measured by the quality of lives preserved or restored; and by the quality of the dying of those in whose interest it is to die; and by the quality of human relationships involved in each death.[12]

This suggests that the success of the ICU relates to a broader remit than the sum total of the survival of individual patients. If this philosophy is supported, then futile care, in the net benefit sense, ought not to be provided: but this will mean that some of the benefits to be assessed relate to the quality of dying, and of relationships, not only to the medical benefits that treatment affords the patient.

To summarize, some conflicts have been identified between parties involved in treatment provision in the ICU, which impact on the use of scarce resources. These conflicts arise from the more general problems of:

- The uncertainties of clinical prognosis where we may have different attitudes to risk.

- The medical tradition of judging treatment to be appropriate or inappropriate raising the problem of defining 'futile' treatment, and the question of 'medical benefit' versus net benefit.

- The weighing of benefits and burdens and the question of who is the best overall judge.

3. Resolving difficult choices

Deciding on the most appropriate treatment involves the weighing of values and ethical concerns as well as the purely medical or evidential considerations. One model which can be helpful in resolving some of the issues discussed, and helpful also in the clinical context, is to develop an ordered approach to the different considerations, as follows:[13]

(1) medical indications;

(2) patient autonomy;

(3) patient's best interests; and

(4) external factors.

Ethical defence of such an approach is necessary because the priorities it entails imply that a decision (e.g. to withdraw mechanical ventilation) which is made at one level does not need to be additionally supported by decisions at successive levels. So, certain medical indications may take precedence over patient autonomy, which in turn takes precedence over the patient's best interests, and so on. If each consideration were seen as being *prima facie* only, it would not be possible to think clearly about the inevitable conflicts in advance of difficult clinical situations.

Conflict between autonomous desires and the collective interest is inevitable. The guidelines developed by the Appleton International Conference[14] suggest this conflict will require at times, 'more than voluntary adjustment': 'the health-care system of any society must have in place a fair and reliable mechanism to explain openly and to enforce justly such adjustments'. One way of approaching such a remit is not to take the *prima facie* path, which may lead us at best to a certain intuitionism and at worst to an unhealthy casuistry, but to proceed using the suggested model of an ethically defensible hierarchy of considerations.

One possible defence of the decisions entailed in such a model is as follows, although there are, of course, alternatives. In a rational and fair allocation of resources decisions must be consistent, and the suggested approach can help to ensure this is so.

1. *Medical indications.* The foremost consideration in whether to provide intensive care must be medical, on the grounds that if a treatment is *not* medically indicated there is no obligation on the part of the doctor to provide it.

2. *Patient autonomy.* The principle of respect for autonomy is central to health care ethics. But if treatment is requested which is not medically indicated autonomy can be justifiably overridden, because there can be no right to demand inappropriate treatment. However, informed and competent patients retain the right to refuse treatment, even where medically indicated.

3. *Patient's best interests.* The third level of decision-making takes the patient's best interests into account. His or her own autonomous wishes should always override such best interests (otherwise autonomy is not being respected). However, where the patient is incompetent, the wishes of the relatives (proxies) will be secondary to the patient's own best interests. This serves to protect the patient.

4. *External factors.* These include the impact of decisions on relatives, their wishes, and resource allocation issues, such as among specialties and hospitals. All of these will jostle for position here, but need be considered only when consideration of the first three levels is not sufficiently directive. The question of whether the impact of decisions on those in competition for resources, and cost factors, properly falls under this heading will be discussed in the following section.

The idea that society may limit the rights of its individual members, such as by withholding health care resources, does not necessarily mean that the rights of the individual are no longer paramount. Such a move is of course justifiable by utilitarian arguments, the well-being of society taking precedence over that of the individual. However, one can also see that the individual can confer certain rights on to the collective, surrendering them, so to speak, in order that that individual may participate in the benefits generated by living in society. This would allow restricting the availability of certain health resources (even to particular individuals), while at the same time the rights of the individual remain paramount in a fundamental sense. This requires the question of 'who decides' with respect to restrictions of access to care to be answered in a democratic way, or at least to be answerable to the democratic process.

4. Competing needs

There is a temptation to place all decisions relating to allocation of intensive care resources under the last consideration: *external factors.* Yet there are strong reasons for considering at least some aspects of these decisions under the first consideration (*medical indications*). This approach is consistent with the view that medical responsibility should consider the needs of the individual patient in the context of society's rights and needs, and in fact is the only approach which can satisfactorily resolve the resource allocation issue at the individual level, while remaining sensitive to the competing needs of other patients.

Guidelines in the medical ethics literature generally indicate that decisions should be based on the benefits and burdens for particular patients, not on social considerations. In other words, it is appropriate to withhold or withdraw treatment on the grounds that there is little likelihood of 'significant therapeutic benefit'[15] for the patient, but not appropriate to base the decision on a productivity oriented perspective (involving a waste of potentially useful resources).

Consider the often-cited dilemma where two patients are in competition for the same resource, the intensive care bed. If care is discontinued for one patient on the grounds that the medical benefit criterion is no longer fulfilled, then treatment can ethically be withdrawn: the patient 'waiting in the wings' need not be referred to at all in justifying the decision. The strict test here would be whether withdrawal of treatment was confined to cases where it still would have been withdrawn even were there no competition for resources. The point is whether the defence of withdrawal of treatment has to resort to the argument from productivity.

A further reason for basing withdrawal of treatment on the medical benefit criterion relates to the group of patients who are borderline, in that only a trial in intensive care will determine whether or not they may benefit from intensive treatment. Because it is often difficult to discontinue treatment once it is begun, this may militate against it being initiated in the first instance, with consequent loss of benefit to some patients in the group. Clear medical benefit criteria will help direct decisions to discontinue inappropriate treatment.

If a limited interpretation of the medical benefit criterion is adopted, there are cases where it may *fail* to resolve the question of the moral acceptability of withdrawing treatment from a patient, for example when there is a patient who would benefit more from the same resource than the patient already undergoing treatment. Where two patients have similar needs for care, and treating one means denying treatment to the other, it has been argued that 'consideration of the opportunity cost of that decision is an appropriate ethical concern'.[14] This is consistent with the goals of justice and efficiency, where efficiency is an expression of the principles of beneficence and non-maleficence. The aphorism, 'it is unethical to be inefficient' explains this, because wasting resources in one area deprives other needy patients who could have benefited from care.

These considerations could be seen as external factors, where resource allocation decisions are to be determined by some developed theory of just distribution. Alternatively, they could be seen to be part and parcel of the medical indications to be considered first, within the context of whether intensive care for a patient is *appropriate*. The fundamental question in resolving such dilemmas is which treatments are appropriate, and which are inappropriate. The question of justice is highly relevant, and often not sufficiently addressed, especially the perspective of whether the cost of any particular distribution of resources is too high—or unfair—for others to bear.

Such reasoning suggests that there are situations where it may be ethically acceptable to withdraw treatment from a patient who could still benefit from care, in order to treat a second patient who would receive greater benefit. The productivity argument which underpins this is that more patients are able to be kept alive or have their lives prolonged. (Note that this relies on an interpretation of 'need' which embraces a patient's 'capacity to benefit' from treatment.) Being a consequentialist rationale, these gains must be weighed against the general dissatisfaction caused by withdrawing treatment from some patients for this reason.[16]

How does such an approach sit with the view that it is unethical to kill an innocent person in order to save another?[17] This will depend on the extent to which withdrawal of treatment is considered to constitute active killing. A number of cases have been adjudicated in the US, where, with few exceptions, the ruling from the courts is that withholding or withdrawing treatment is legally acceptable[18] where the burdens attendant on the treatment outweigh the benefits to the patient. The withdrawal of advanced life support has been treated in the same manner as the question of withdrawal of nutrition and hydration from incompetent patients, in the three states where courts have addressed these issues.[19] The view is that 'switching off' a ventilator or 'pulling the plug' is ethically no different from discontinuing any inappropriate medical treatment.[20] The question of whether withdrawal of treatment is ethical or not seems to rest on whether it is appropriate (in terms of whether we value what it is *for*), rather than on the nature of the act itself.

In the UK the relevant judgement in this respect is the Bland case,[21] where it was ruled that despite the inability of the defendant to consent, the physicians, 'may lawfully discontinue all life-sustaining treatment and medical supportive measures designed to keep the defendant alive'.[22] The relevance of this case to the present discussion rests on the discontinuance of life support being properly categorized as an ommission, and no different from not initiating life support in the first place. In such cases the doctor, in discontinuing life support, is allowing the patient to die of their pre-existing condition: 'the doctor is simply allowing his patient to die in the sense that he is desisting from taking a step which might, in certain circumstances, prevent his patient from dying as a result of his pre-existing condition'.[22]

Such reasoning, although itself not without its critics,[23] suggests that withdrawing treatment when it is still needed may be no different ethically from not initiating needed care in the first place. Under scarcity, this latter course of action may be justified; so that the description of the situation where two patients compete for the same resource as, 'killing an innocent person in order to save another' is misleading. Rather than the question being the emotional one of, 'should a doctor be entitled to switch a life support system off or pull the plug?[24] it becomes one of whether the doctor should or should not continue to provide the patient with medical treatment, which if continued will prolong the patient's life.

In this alternative phrasing of the question there is more leeway for the doctor to assess the needs of the individual patient in the context of societal interests, and also for the notion of opportunity cost to enter in (in this case being those benefits foregone by the patient who would receive greater benefit from the treatment). Justice requires that resources are not wasted on patients whom they cannot help. The principle of utility—and some would argue of justice also—requires that they are used preferentially for those patients whom they can help the most. These requirements must also, of course, be balanced against other *prima facie* principles, for instance, that which underpins the duty of the doctor to maintain the fiduciary relationship with the patient. However, no one principle is absolute, allowing scope for judging it ethical in certain cases to withdraw treatment from one patient in order to treat another. Much, as always in applied ethics, will depend on the particular case, and the discrepancy in the size of benefits to be conferred on the respective patients competing for resources. Much will also depend on the management of the patients and their relatives, good communication, and whether emotional support and assurance is forthcoming to both the relatives and members of the health care team.

Patients' and relatives' wishes are always relevant, but may not always be determinative. For justice also requires that patients' and their relatives' sanction the transfer of resources to others: either when they themselves can no longer benefit from them, or even when benefit to them is disproportionately less than benefit to others. These are examples of conflict between autonomous desires and the collective interest which may well require, 'more than voluntary adjustment',[25] and where the attending doctors have an obligation to facilitate these unpalatable choices, resulting from their having duties to more than simply the patient before them.

5. Conclusion

Thus, there are certain kinds of allocative decisions, between patients competing for intensive care resources, which are properly addressed under the first head of *medical indications*. This is to interpret *medical indications* such that the entailed value judgements are acknowledged as not only unavoidable, but also as contributory to the final ethical choice in the way the resources are distributed:

The ethically responsive doctor will thus find himself more and more involved in social and individual ethical issues, impelled to act responsibly in both spheres.[26]

Admittedly, there is a fine distinction to be drawn between the doctor serving as such an expert witness and being laid open to the charge of trying to conceal social decisions behind the cloak of clinical practice. But who is better placed to raise the matter of painful choices and inform the public debate?

Nevertheless, there are many resource allocation decisions falling under the head of *external factors*, which relate to the broader issues and compromises which affect the ICU. Budgetary limits and institutional constraints involve decisions which cannot justly be made on a case-by-case basis. These must be addressed as a matter of public policy.[27] Such policies need to be formulated, and, through open discussion and debate, set realistic and humane standards of intensive care. As recommended by the Appleton International Conference, it is also critical that there be widespread dissemination of such principles and guidelines to decision-makers at all levels, and to the general public, and that this should be routine.[25]

Notes

1. Luce, J.M. (1990). Ethical principles in critical Care. *Journal of the American Medical Association*, **263**, 696–700; 699.
2. Veatch, R.M. and Spicer, C.M. (1992). Medically futile care: The role of the physician in setting limits. *American Journal of Law and Medicine*, **XVIII**, 15–36; 15.
3. Stanley, J. (Guest Editor) (1992). The Appleton International Conference: Developing guidelines for decisions to forgo life-prolonging medical treatment. *Journal of Medical Ethics*, **18** (Suppl.), 6–7.
4. Note 3, p. 8.
5. Note 2, p. 23.
6. Tomlinson, T. and Brody, H. (1988). Ethics and communication in do-not-resuscitate orders. *New England Journal of Medicine*, **318**, 43–46; 43.
7. Note 2, p. 28.
8. McCling, J.A. and Kamer, R.S. (1990). Legislating ethics: Implications of New York's do-Not-resuscitate Law. *New England Journal of Medicine*, **323**, 270–2; 270.
9. Fisher, M.M. and Raper, R.F. (1990). Withdrawing and withholding treatment in intensive care *The Medical Journal of Australia*, **153**, 217–25; 218.
10. Brannigan, M. (1993). Oregon's experiment. *Health Care Analysis*, **1**, 15–32. Oregon Health Services Commission (1991). *Prioritization of health services: A report to the Governor and Legislature*.
11. Honigsbaum, F. (1992). Who shall live? Who shall die?—Oregon's health financing proposals. *King's Fund College Papers* 4, King's College Fund, 2 Palace Court, London W2 4HS. Dixon, J. and Welch, H.G. (1992). Priority setting: lessons from Oregon, *Lancet*, **337**, 891–4. Klein, R. (1991). On the Oregon trail: rationing health care. *British Medical Journal*, **302**, 1–2.

12. Dunstan, G.R. (1985). Hard questions in intensive care. *Anaesthesia*, **40**, 479–82.
13. Schneiderman, L.J. and Spragg, R.G. (1988). Ethical decisions in discontinuing mechanical ventilation. *New England Journal of Medicine*, **318**, 984–8; 985.
14. Note 3, p. 18.
15. Kilner, J.F. (1990). *Who lives? Who dies? Ethical criteria in patient selection*, p. 120. Yale University Press, New Haven.
16. Note 15, p. 128.
17. Note 15, p. 129.
18. Landmark cases are: *In re Quinlan* (NJ 1976); *Brophy* v. *New England Sinai Hospital, Inc* (Mass 1986).
19. Ruark, J.E. and Raffin, T.A. (1988). Initiating and withdrawing life support: Principles and practice in adult medicine. *New England Journal of Medicine*, **318**, 25–30; 30.
20. *Barber* v. *Los Angeles County Superior Court* (Cal 1983).
21. *Airedale NHS Trust* (Respondents) v. *Bland* (Acting by his Guardian ad litem) (Appellant) Judgment: 4 February 1993 House of Lords.
22. Note 21, p. 12.
23. Finnis, J.M. (1993). *Bland*: Crossing the Rubicon? Draft paper. Published in the *Law Quarterly Review*.
24. Note 21, p. 14.
25. Note 3, p. 18.
26. Pellegrino, E.D. (1979). *Humanism and the physician*, (1st edn). University of Tennessee Press.
27. Note 13, p. 988.

13
A Theological Overview

G.R. Dunstan

1. Theology and medical ethics

In a book concerned with the law and ethics of medical practice, what is the function of a 'theological overview'? For the purpose of this chapter, theology may be said to be the study or understanding of God and his relation to the created order, and of man's place in it. (In this chapter, as in standard English, when 'man' is required in a species-specific sense, as in *Homo sapiens*, it will be so used, and with the common pronoun. When a gender-specific sense is required, *mas, femina*, the distinction will be drawn.) A theology so described entails certain doctrines about man's own nature and destiny, and so of his duties.

Even this statement, in its simplicity, betrays its origin in a culture which assumes a relation between God, man, and creation not evident in some other religions. The formative theology in Western culture and ethics is generally spoken of as Judaeo-Christian. Its basic material is quarried from the writings or texts, accumulated and declared sacred by the communities, first Jewish then Christian, which produced them. They are now called the Old Testament and the New. There are still many people who assume that ethical questions, as they arise, can be answered by appeal to these Scriptures. In Islamic societies, the Qur'ān is appealed to in the same way, and with much skill and ingenuity.[1] To this, two things must be said in reply.

First, it is evident, after but little thought, that the complex questions thrown up by our contemporary scientific and technological culture cannot be resolved by direct appeal to texts written in ancient cultures where those questions could not arise. A theological ethics cannot be equated with, or restricted to, a detailed prescriptive appeal to scriptures, as though the Bible could 'tell us what to do'. That would be to do violence to the Scriptures and the purposes for which they were written.

Secondly, theology is a wider discipline than biblical studies. Theology is the product of a tradition of reflection, in which given beliefs are re-formulated in the light of philosophies and ideologies dominant at particular times, particularly those of the Greeks. Platonism, with its dualist distinction between matter and spirit, body and soul, became a major influence on the formation of theology and ethics, particularly with the commanding authority of St. Augustine in the last centuries of the Roman empire. In the twelfth and thirteenth centuries, European philosophers and theologians, thanks to Arab scholars and commentators, rediscovered a lost Aristotle. In a magnificent intellectual achievement, they reinterpreted the received theology into the thought forms of Aristotle, now synthesized with an Augustinian Platonism.

That achievement, the work largely of Roger Bacon, Albert of Cologne, and his pupil, St. Thomas Aquinas, first enabled the rebirth of the natural sciences which we now associate with the Renaissance. Secondly, it gave us grounds on which to articulate an ethics of practice appropriate to the developing science and technology of our day. It could do this because both science and ethics were grounded in reason, both products of the rational nature of man.

From Aristotle, these scholastics took an understanding of man as by nature rational and social. From the theological tradition, they held that man was made in the image of God, the creator and the Father of all mankind. Man, therefore, was truly responding to God when he searched out by his rationality the hidden ways of nature and, as a social being, applied his knowledge benevolently to human need. Roger Bacon wrote of what remedies for defective sight might come from the study of optics. By trial and experiment would come experience, the only way of escape from unquestioning bondage to tradition. Hence, the eclipse of Galen by Vesalius, of Thomas Vicary by William Harvey, and the advance from scientific observation to experimental research. A simple tablet in the Botanic Garden in Oxford carries an inscription, unaccredited, but from Roger Bacon: *sine experientia nihil sufficienter sciri potest* (without trial, experiment, nothing can be sufficiently known).[2]

The ethics were grounded on the same foundation. By moral reasoning, we are to establish, in particular instances of claim, particular duties: what virtue obliges us to do; what each owes to the other and is owed in a structured society.[3] Man is also a social being (*zoon politikon*), and the good consists in fulfilling the end (*telos*) to which his humanity, rational and social, naturally aspires. Theology carried that aspiration beyond terrestrial, human society, towards God himself: man is made for fellowship with God and to enjoy him in his eternity. To natural virtue there were added, therefore, the theological virtues; and we owe to one another not only our service to meet bodily and social need but also service of such a sort that in giving it we advance also the capacity for ultimate fulfilment. Religious people sometimes call this 'the spiritual dimension' and fear for its neglect in modern medicine.

The object of medical concern, therefore, is not simply the vulnerable body, but man, served through the body. The duty of care, in its true character, is governed by respect for this embodied humanity in its integral worth and destiny (*caritas*). A mutual human duty is refined in medicine into a professional duty, shaped, developed, and transmitted by corporate practice in succeeding generations.[4]

2. Moral reasoning

A theological overview, therefore, gives us an ethics of practice derived from philosophy and theology, mutually interpreted.[5] Philosophy and theology had been married in church, so to speak, by St Paul. In a crucial passage in the first two chapters of his Epistle to the Romans, he recognized that the Greeks (Gentiles), although not taught to discern good and evil by the Mosaic law as the Jews were, could 'do by nature the things of the law'—could recognize that distinction in their own consciences; by reason they could learn the truth and goodness of God from the evidences of his divinity seen in creation. The 'Gentile conscience', as it came to be called, is the common faculty which enables adherents of different faiths, or of none, to agree on international conventions, like those of Geneva, for the just conduct of war and the protection of prisoners, and those of Helsinki and of the World Health Organization for the conduct of medical practice and research.

It would follow that when we turn to the ethics of particular medical interventions, like those assigned to this chapter, no 'answers' can or need be read off from sacred scriptures. Ethics is the product of moral reasoning on the facts of the case in the light of principles, derived from religion and philosophy, and established in the conscience of 'the educated moral agent' 'acting on the basis of a true and rational judgement'.[6]

That judgement, the outcome of moral reasoning, is not exercised in each case in isolation as though there were no moral continuity in practice. The exercise is undertaken within a moral community, a society held together by a sufficient number of inherited common beliefs, presumptions, and practices. Medical ethics, therefore, concerns itself not only with practice but also with relationship. When the ethical relationship, which some, following Rousseau, call the contract, between doctors and the public breaks down, not only is practice put in jeopardy—and with it medical and nursing staff—but also moral reasoning becomes more inconclusive and contentious.

A classic example of the problems facing medicine and its ethics arises in some cases concerning handicapped neonates and those who are at the end of their lives or are in persistent vegetative conditions. For these individuals, the capacities of medicine to prolong existence may be in tension with the non-technical and more basic presumptions concerning how the individual must or should be treated.[7] Most acutely, this may arise when the question arises whether or not basic care, in the form of nutrition and hydration, should or must be provided.

3. Nutrition and hydration

To provide food and drink is a natural duty, one proper to human nature, owed to man and beast. It is enjoined also by the strict commands of religion, inscribed in sacred texts: 'Deal thy bread to the hungry . . . hide not thyself from thine own flesh' (*Isaiah* 58:7); 'If thine enemy hunger, feed him; if he thirst, give him drink' (*Romans* 12:20). The assurance of a diet adequate for nutrition is therefore a proper part of medical care, the professional refinement of a common human obligation. Sometimes, it is the medical duty to provide it by nasogastric or intravenous infusion, when the body cannot take nourishment or fluid unaided, as, for instance, in intensive or terminal care.

But is the duty absolute, one to be discharged without exception; without regard to consequence or circumstance? What if the body cannot tolerate nutrition, however administered, and irremediable gastrointestinal or renal disturbance or failure follow? It would cease then to be in the patient's interest to infuse nutrition—unless the rejection were predictably temporary with a good prognosis beyond. It might even be necessary to withdraw hydration and rely on oral nursing care. The clinician must reason his or her way to a decision apt to each patient, given the indications for each, and compatible with reliable professional opinion. Given that the leading criterion is the best interest of the patient, a doctor who felt bound by his or her religion not to withdraw, regardless of consequence, would face an ethical crisis, a conflict between personal and professional conscience. The duty to feed is presumptive, not absolute. The presumption in favour of nutrition is rebuttable for grave cause relating to the patient's interest.

To withdraw nutrition is not to abandon the patient, not to 'leave him to die'. It is to attune the treatment, the management, to suit the patient's condition. The duty of care continues, exercised in palliative medicine, including relief of discomfort, pain, distress, until the body systems fail and the patient dies. For some, this is merely an argument in justification of euthanasia (albeit in a passive form). Not so: the slogan 'passive euthanasia' distorts reality, as most slogans do. Palliative care is active, skilled. It does not kill the patient; it serves his or her interest in dying a peaceful natural death.

English law now forbids the forcible feeding of hunger strikers. This is not grounded on a tacit recognition of a supposed 'right' to commit suicide. (Suicide is a liberty, not a right.) It is grounded on the principle of respect for bodily integrity and self-determination. To administer medical treatment to an adult who is conscious and of sound mind, without consent, constitutes a tort/delict (a civil wrong) and the crime of battery/assault—except, under necessity, in emergency. Under the Mental Health Act 1983, for example, doctors may override a psychiatric patient's refusal of food in certain circumstances. But in October 1993, the English Court of Appeal overruled an earlier High Court decision in which a single judge authorized the forcible feeding of a psychiatric patient suffering from *anorexia nervosa*. In the earlier proceedings, which had been for a temporary declaration only, the patient had not been represented, so her right to refuse consent had not been argued.[8]

The duty to feed, then, is not absolute. It is presumptive, rebuttable in certain circumstances, including a patient's refusal of consent. For some patients, however, the issue of consent is in itself problematic and their management much more complex. A patient in a persistent vegetative state (PVS), having suffered the destruction of the cerebral cortex, is in no position to give consent or to withhold it. Unlike the patient who is brainstem dead, the PVS patient has still sufficient function in the brainstem to sustain heart-beat and respiration so long as sufficient nutrient fluid is supplied. In the case of *Airedale NHS Trust* v. *Bland*,[9] the House of Lords held that it was not unlawful for doctors to withdraw life-supporting medical treatment, including artificial feeding through a nasogastric tube, from such a patient who had no prospect of any recovery or improvement, when it was known that the discontinuance of treatment would cause the patient's death within a matter of weeks.

Mr Anthony Bland, at the age of 17, had been crushed in the Hillsborough stadium disaster and had been cared for medically for over three years in the persistent vegetative state. He was completely insensate and there was no medical prospect of recovery. His doctors, with the full agreement of his parents, wished to withdraw the means of intensive care. The Airedale NHS Trust obtained from the Family Division of the High Court (Sir Stephen Brown, President) a declaration that such an action would not be unlawful. This was confirmed in the Court of Appeal. The Solicitor-General, acting as guardian *ad litem* for Mr Bland, appealed to the House of Lords. The five judgments dismissing the appeal are a monument of medico-ethical legal reasoning.

In upholding the declaration, which enabled artificial feeding to be withdrawn without threat of criminal or civil proceedings, the structure of the argument was finely drawn. Artificial feeding was professionally regarded as a form of medical treatment, 'and even if it is not strictly medical treatment, it must form part of the medical care of the patient'.[10] If that treatment were withdrawn, the patient would die. Since what was sought in the Court was a declaration that the withdrawal contemplated would not be unlawful, it was important that the action be not interpreted as one for the direct killing of the patient; for that in law would be no other than murder or manslaughter. So, the cessation of nourishment and hydration would be an omission, not an act: an omission which would not be criminal unless the doctors were under a present duty to continue the regime. Were they under that duty? The decision to mount the regime was taken when Mr Bland came into the doctors' care, in no condition to consent to it. Under the principle of emergency, it was held to be in his best interest that he should be supported in this way in the hope—not then impossible—that he might recover. When all hope of recovery had been abandoned, his interest in being kept alive had disappeared, and with it the justification for a continued intervention on his body without consent. The duty to maintain nutrition and hydration had therefore ceased: the omission would not, therefore, be a criminal act, and the declaration sought could be made.

The ethical nuances in the judgment are important. Their Lordships were careful to avoid pronouncing as lawful an action intended to end life, even though life would end as a consequence of the not unlawful withdrawal. They refused also to declare the termination of Mr Bland's life as in his best interest: in his persistent insensate state, he had no interests either in living or in dying. The state has an interest, protected by the law, in maintaining the principle of the sanctity of human life—even though it is not absolute, being set in tension with the principle of self-determination which underlies the necessity of consent. For this reason, they declared that, for the immediate future, all such cases should be brought before the Court, partly to assure that they fell within the terms of the present declaration, partly to protect doctors in the exercise of their professional duty and discretion. The assurances required by the Ethics Committee of the British Medical Association (BMA) in its *Discussion Paper on Treatment of Patients in Persistent Vegetative State*[11] were to be followed. Doctors so acting could feel reasonably assured that they carried with them a responsible and competent body of professional opinion, so as to satisfy the test outlined in the case of *Bolam* v. *Friern Hospital Management Committee*[12] of reasonable professional conduct.

The question of whether and when artificial feeding may be withdrawn has been expounded here in terms of the common law. The ethics of the question have not, however, been ignored. They are acknowledged, in the Bland judgment, as being prior to the questions of law. The ethics are not only in statements of principle—the tension between respect for self-determination and respect for the sanctity of life; they are the ethics of professional practice also. Lord Goff, for example, was explicit in affirming the primary responsibility of the doctor for decision; the law is both the framework within which he must decide and the protector of his liberty and duty of discretion in decision. These are his words, following a favourable comment on the BMA discussion paper on the treatment of PVS patients:

I also feel that those who are concerned that a matter of life and death, such as is involved in a decision to withhold life support in a case of this kind, should be left to the doctors would do well to study this paper. The truth is that, in the course of their work, doctors frequently have to make decisions which may affect the continued survival of their patients, and are in reality far more experienced in matters of this kind than are the judges. It is nevertheless the function of the judges to state the legal principles upon which the lawfulness of the actions of doctors depend; but in the end the decisions to be made in individual cases must rest with the doctors themselves. In these circumstances, what is required is a sensitive understanding by both the judges and the doctors of each other's respective functions, and in particular a determination by the judges not merely to understand the problems facing the medical profession in cases of this kind, but also to regard their professional standards with respect. Mutual understanding between the doctors and the judges is the best way to ensure the evolution of a sensitive and sensible legal framework for the treatment and care of patients, with a sound ethical base, in the interests of the patients themselves.[13]

4. Should all patients be treated?

This is the second question considered in this chapter, and it must be refined before it can be answered.

Since health, in the sense of physical and mental well-being, is a product of good natural function, we all have an interest in its pursuit and a natural claim on means available to correct or alleviate malfunction. We have also a natural duty to serve that interest, when we can, in our fellows. Parents have a particular duty towards their children. Doctors, professing knowledge and skills proper to health care, owe a professional duty towards their patients. The nature of the claim on professional duty varies with varieties of social and economic organization, and of resources available. The UK, under the National Health Service Acts, has conferred on all its subjects, and on some others, a statutory right to medical care (i.e. to consultation and advice and to such treatment as is medically indicated and available). It does not confer a right to any particular treatment of the patient's choosing against medical advice.

The object of treatment is to serve the patient's interest in health and life, by means appropriate and proportionate at every stage. It does not oblige a doctor to futility, that is, to continue supposedly curative intervention beyond the point when the condition has become incurable—that would be adverse to the patient's interest. The medical duty at that point is not to abandon treatment but to change it, to palliative and, when necessary, terminal care. Neither does it, in the general philosophy of medicine, entail an absolute duty to strive to keep alive. Good clinical practice recognizes a time to die and serves the patient's interest in dying. Treatment is best decided, when possible, after consultation with the patient, with relatives, and nursing and medical staff. But responsibility for the treatment chosen rests with the clinician in charge. British law refuses to take that responsibility from him.

In the UK, the guardian of patients' rights and of doctors' responsibilities is the common law, developed by judges in the courts. Courts do not *order* particular treatment; they *authorize* whatever treatment or withholding of treatment is chosen by competent medical opinion to be in the patient's best interests. The medical duty is exercised within a legal liberty. Two recent cases bring out the ethical principle involved.

The baby *J* was born prematurely at 21 weeks' gestation, was resuscitated and placed on a ventilator for a month, and afterwards, episodically, according to need. He was severely brain damaged, blind, probably deaf, subject to convulsions, probably never able to speak or develop intellectually, yet able to feel pain. His life expectancy might be into his late 'teens. The child was a ward of court. It fell to the court, therefore, as *parens patriae*, to exercise the normal parental function of consent, as to whether the baby should be returned to the respirator on the next occasion of need. The doctors in charge thought it was inappropriate to do so. The judge withheld the court's consent. On behalf of the Official Solicitor, it was submitted on appeal that consent could never be withheld from treatment which would enable a child to survive, whatever the pain or side-effects, and whatever the quality of life thereafter.

The Court of Appeal[14] rejected this 'absolutist' approach. 'In real life there are presumptions, strong presumptions and almost overwhelming presumptions, but there are few, if any, absolutes'.[15] 'There is a strong presumption in favour of action which would prolong life, but it is not irrebuttable'.[16] The first and paramount consideration of the Court should be the interests of the ward. If it would not be in the interests of the ward to subject it to treatment which would cause increased suffering and produce no commensurable benefit, the court would be justified in refusing consent. The appeal was dismissed.

The second case demonstrated even more forcibly the locus of responsibility. The baby W suffered brain damage in a fall when a month old. At 18 months he was severely microcephalic, he had severe cerebral palsy and epilepsy, and cortical blindness. He was fed by a nasogastric tube. Unanimous medical opinion was that he would not develop beyond his present state of functioning, but that this might deteriorate. Life expectancy was short. None of the medical evidence presented to the court favoured mechanical ventilation, should a life-threatening event occur. In this, the consultant in charge was supported by the health authority and the Official Solicitor. However, the mother and the local authority (the child having been placed by it with foster parents) sought an order to compel the health authority to provide all available treatment, including intensive resuscitation. The judge granted an interim injunction to that effect on the ground that it served the child's best interest and the interest of justice. The health authority appealed, now with the support of the local authority. The mother opposed the appeal.

In the Court of Appeal,[17] the Master of the Rolls declared that, 'the fundamental issue was whether the Court in the exercise of its inherent power to protect the interests of a minor child could ever require a medical practitioner to adopt a course of treatment which, in the *bona fide* clinical judgment of the practitioner, was contra-indicated as not being in the patient's best interests' ... 'His Lordship could not, at present, conceive of any circumstances in which that would be other than an abuse of power as directly or indirectly requiring the practitioner to act contrary to the fundamental duty he owed to his patient'.[18] The court set aside the judge's order, so leaving the health authority and its medical staff free, subject to consent not being withdrawn, to treat baby W in accordance with their best clinical judgement.

Clinical responsibility is an ethical responsibility, of which the medical practitioner is the moral agent.[19] Is there a risk in this that clinical judgement may be clouded by personal prejudice or by religious scruple? Indeed, in the Bland case, Lord Browne-Wilkinson mentioned evidence that 'the Roman Catholic church and orthodox Jews are opposed'[20] to withdrawal of life support in the present case. Rabbinic Judaism, as expounded by Lord Jakobovits, the former Chief Rabbi, a recognized authority on Jewish medical ethics, might well oppose withdrawal because of Jewish doctrine that every moment of human life is infinitely precious, and so active treatment to prolong life must be given until the process of dying had actually begun.[21] For a Jewish doctor and family, both within the orthodox community, that doctrine might well determine their mutual expectations of care. (In other sections of Judaism, variously called Liberal or Reform, it might not.) But with a patient outside the community, whose family did not share that conviction, the doctor could not persist without consent: he must be guided by the corporate conscience of his profession as to what was acceptable and required practice; or commit the patient's care into other hands.

As for Roman Catholics, there is reason to question whether the evidence to which the Lord Justice referred was representative of magisterial teaching. A distinguished English Roman Catholic moralist, Fr. Kevin Kelly, in a reasoned paper,[22] cites both an established tradition and contemporary authorities to argue that the artificial feeding was what moralists call an 'extraordinary', or optional, procedure which might licitly be withdrawn, and that, 'this should not, from an ethical point of view, be regarded as killing by starvation'.[23] And well he might so conclude. For, on 24 November 1957, Pope Pius XII, in an allocution to Catholic anaesthetists, declared artificial life support by ventilator to be an 'extraordinary' means which the patient was not bound to request nor doctors to administer. After sufficient trial, it was licit to withdraw the ventilator before circulation had ceased.[24] 'Pro-life' activists might decline to extend this doctrine to the persistent vegetative state, which was not in 1957 distinguished as such; but competent Catholic moralists have no difficulty in finding consistency with the tradition.

A short answer can now be given to the last question posed in this chapter: Should all patients be treated? All patients should be received, respected, and heard. All patients should be advised, on the basis of information available, diagnosis, prognosis, possibility, uncertainty, doubt. All should be offered treatment, if called for, apt to their condition and if available. None can oblige a doctor to offer treatment against his judgement of what is in the patient's best interest. A doctor so receiving a patient and acting in a manner defensible by his professional peers and with the consent of the patient properly informed, enjoys the protection of the law. The ethics are not an ethics of act only, but also of relationship: one between the doctor, the patient, society, and the law. The law is the protector of the common good, as faith, philosophy and ethics are, over time, its creator.

Notes

1. Albar, Mohammed Ali (1986). *Human development as revealed in the Holy Qur'ān and Hadith: The creation of man between medicine and the Qur'ān.* Saudi Publishing and Distributing House, Jeddah. The author, MRCP, DM, MB, BGH, is Consultant in Islamic Medicine, King Fahad Medical Research Center, King Abdul Aziz University, Jeddah. This is a basic textbook (149

pp.) on embryology, illustrated like any modern textbook. The contemporary science is presented as 'Corroboration of scientific truths in the Holy Qur'ān and Hadīth' (p. 9).

2. Crombie, A.C. (1953) *Robert Grosseteste and the origins of experimental science in Oxford*. Clarendon Press, Oxford. The quotation is from Roger Bacon's *Opus Maius*, VI.I. It occurs, translated in a long footnote extract, on p. 141.

3. MacIntyre, A. (1981). *After virtue: A study in moral theory*, p. 115 Duckworth, London.

4. Note 3, pp. 174ff.

5. Byrne, P. (1992). *The philosophical and theological foundation of ethics: An introduction to moral theory*. Macmillan, Basingstoke; St. Martin's Press, New York,

6. Note 3, p. 40.

7. See Chapters 2 and 8.

8. *Re J* [1992] 4 All ER 614.

9. *Airedale NHS Trust* v. *Bland* [1993] 1 All ER 821.

10. Per Lord Goff, p. 871 in note 9.

11. BMA (British Medical Association) (1992, September). *Consultation on treatment of patients in persistent vegetative state*. Circulated for comment by the BMA Ethics Committee.

12. [1957] 2 All ER 118.

13. Note 10, p. 872.

14. *Re J (a minor) (wardship: medical treatment)* [1990] 3 All ER 930.

15. Per Lord Donaldson, p. 937 in note 14.

16. Per Lord Donaldson, p. 938 in note 14.

17. *Re W (a minor) (refusal of treatment)* [1992] 3 WLR 758.

18. *The Times* Law Report, 12 June 1992.

19. Dunstan, G.R., (1989). The doctor as responsible moral agent. In *Doctors' decisions: Ethical conflicts in medical practice*, (ed. G.R. Dunstan and E.A. Shinebourne), Oxford University Press.

20. Per Lord Browne-Wilkinson, p. 879 in note 9.

21. Jakobovits, I. (1983). The doctor's duty to heal and the patient's consent. In *Consent in medicine: Convergence and divergence in tradition*, (ed. G.R. Dunstan and M.J. Seller), pp. 32–6. King Edward's Hospital Fund for London. Jakobovits, I. (1991). 'The hospice movement from the Jewish point of view. In Byrne, P. *et al.*, Hospice Care: Jewish reservations considered in a comparative Ethical Study, *Palliative Medicine*, 5, 187–200. See also, Schostak, Rabbi Z. (1994). Jewish ethical guidelines for resuscitation and artificial nutrition and hydration of the dying elderly. *Journal of Medical Ethics*, 20, 93–100.

22. Kelly, K. (1993). Rest for Tony Bland. *The Tablet*, 13 March, 323–33.

23. Note 21, p. 323.

24. Duncan, A.S., Dunstan, G.R., and Welbourn, R.B. (ed.) (1981). *Dictionary of medical ethics*, at Life, Prolongation of, (pp. 226–8). Darton, Longman & Todd, London and Crossroad, New York.

Index